Veterinary Surgery
A Practical Guide

The Authors

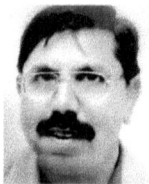

Dr. P.B. Patel, graduated in veterinary science from Gujarat Agricultural University in 1987 and joined as Veterinary Officer with in-service post graduate students in same University. He completed his M.V.Sc. in 1990 and Ph.D in 1996 in same University. He is author of more than 50 research papers in national and international journals and more than 25 popular articles and five booklets. He was awarded with five gold medals and best teacher award. He is at present, working as Professor and Head, Department of Veterinary Surgery and Radiology, College of Veterinary Science & Animal Husbandry, Junagadh Agricultural University, Junagadh.

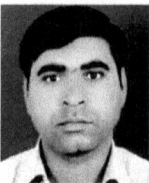

Dr. A.M. Patel received professional degree from Sardar Krushinagar Dantiwada Agricultural University in 2007. He has completed Master degree in Veterinary Surgery and Radiology from Anand Agricultural University in 2009. He worked as Veterinary Officer in Animal Husbandry Department, Gujarat and Panjarapole. He joined Junagadh Agricultural University in 2012 as an Assistant Professor. He is author of 3 international, 8 national, 10 popular articles and 4 booklets.

Veterinary Surgery
A Practical Guide

– Authors –
Dr. P.B. Patel
Dr. A.M. Patel

2016
Daya Publishing House®

A Division of
Astral International Pvt. Ltd.
New Delhi - 110 002

Cataloging in Publication Data--DK
Courtesy: D.K. Agencies (P) Ltd. <docinfo@dkagencies.com>

Patel, P. B., author.
Veterinary surgery : a practical guide / authors, Dr. P.B. Patel, Dr. A.M. Patel.
    pages cm
    ISBN 978-93-5130-927-7 (International Edition)

    1. Veterinary surgery--India.   I. Patel, A. M., author.
II. Title.
SF703.P38 2016   DDC 636.08970954   23

Published by   :   **Daya Publishing House®**
A Division of
Astral International Pvt. Ltd.
– ISO 9001:2008 Certified Company –
4760-61/23, Ansari Road, Darya Ganj
New Delhi-110 002
Ph. 011-43549197, 23278134
E-mail: info@astralint.com
Website: www.astralint.com

Laser Typesetting: SSMG Computer Graphics, Delhi - 110 084

Printed at   :   Replika Press Pvt. Ltd.

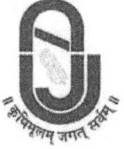

College of Veterinary Science & A. H.
Junagadh Agricultural University
Junagadh- 362 001, Gujarat, India

Dr. P. H. Tank
Principal & Dean
Veterinary college, JAU, Junagadh

Contact: (O) +91-285-2670722
E-mail: covsah@jau.in

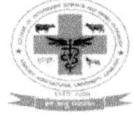

Foreword

A practical guideline for the graduating scholars and field veterinarians in the veterinary professional particularly in the subject of Veterinary Surgery and Radiology was the demand of time since long. The book "Veterinary Surgery – A Practical Guide" fulfills almost all the requirements as per VCI guidelines for the courses pertaining to General Surgery, Anaesthesiology and diagnostic imaging. Authors have also justified the practical view point during clinical surgery based on their rich experience in the clinical fields.

I congratulate both the authors for their keen interest in their field of expertise and to write this book based on their experience and so also expect them to periodically revise the contents as per need in continuing to the fast development of their versatile discipline of the veterinary sciences.

(P.H. Tank)

Preface

A concise practical note as per new Veterinary Council of India syllabus for Veterinary Surgery and Radiology is demand since long from undergraduate students, teachers and field Veterinarians. Non availability of such publication and high cost are constraints for students and field Veterinarians.

As per Veterinary Council of India syllabus the topics are divided in three units i.e. Semesters. We have tried to describe text including many key points and bullet forms with illustrations in very simple language so as digest by students and fields Veterinarians. Dr. P. B. Patel had vast 27 years of academic and field experience and applied his knowledge in each and every point. Dr. A. M. Patel had 5 years of experience in field and three years of experience as teacher.

We always welcome constructive suggestions that will improve the further edition for betterments.

Authors wish to put their appreciation to respective family members for their endurance, constant support and encouragement during writing and acknowledge the facts with love and gratitude.

Every effort has been made to ensure accuracy of the information given in the book. The authors and publisher accept no responsibility for any error or omissions which might have appeared in the book.

Dr. P.B. Patel
Dr. A.M. Patel

Contents

Unit – III

UNIT I

Chapter 1

Surgical Instruments and Equipments

Surgeon should know basic information about instrument like Scalpel, B.P handle, B.P blades, Scissors, Towel clamp, Allis tissue forceps, Thumb forceps, Retractors, Needle holders, Suture needles- traumatic and atraumatic, their shapes and use, Rumenotomy set, Intestinal clamps, different types of mouth gauge (buttler, Vernell, Gray), Eye Spaculum, Hobbels, Tounge forceps, Tooth rasp, Stomach tube, Probang, Endotracheal tubes, Trocar and canula, Trephines, Catheters, Syme's abscess knife, Emasculator, Welping forceps, Teat slitter, Gigli wires saw and handle, Plaster of paris cutter, Bone cutter, Chisel, osteotome, Grooved director, Kirschner hand and key, Bone plates, K wires etc.

Equipments like Hydraulic operation tables, Surgical diathermy, Autoclave, Sterilizer, Boyle's apparatus, Suction apparatus, Surgical electrocautery, Shadow less lamp, X- ray machine and its accessory etc.

Each type of instrument is designed for a particular use and should be used only for that purpose. Use of instruments for procedures for which they are not designed may break or dull the instruments.

The instruments must be used properly and receive routine care and maintenance to prevent corrosion, pitting and discoloration. The instruments should be rinsed in cool water immediately after the surgical procedure to prevent blood, tissue, saline or other foreign matter from dying on them. Instruments should be dried immediately after washing as tap water contains mineral that leads to discoloration of the instruments. Ideally one should use distil or de-ionized water. Delicate instruments should be cleaned and sterilized separately.

Common surgical instruments

a) **Artery forceps:** It is used to arrest the blood during the operative procedure.

b) **Allis tissue forceps:** It is used to hold tissue for better deeper exposure.

c) **Needle holder:** It is used to hold surgical needle during suturing.

d) **Bard- Parker (B.P) handle:** To hold the B.P blade.

e) **B.P blade:** Use for incised the tissue with minimum trauma.

f) **Scissors:** For the dissection of the soft tissue.

g) **Towel clamp:** To grasp and secure the drape.

h) **Suturing needle:** To suture the tissue.

i) **Thumb forceps:** To hold the soft tissue.

Except b.p blade all instrument must be sterilised before use in operation.

Specialized Instruments

1. **Teat surgery:** Teat bistoury, teat slitter, teat scissor, teat tumor extractor, teat siphone, teat infusion tube, teat dilator etc.

2. **Dental instruments:** Tooth cutter, tooth rasper, mouth gauge, tooth nipper, tooth scalar, tooth extractor ctc.

3. **Orthopaedic instruments:** bone holding clamp, owl, K nail, Steinmann pin, rush pin, pin cutter, guide wire, orthopaedic wire, bone cutter, chiseal and hammer, trephine, orthopaedic drill, bone plate, orthopaedic screw, Screw driver, Plier, Filler, plaster cutting saw etc.

4. **Ophthalmic instruments:** Ophthalmoscope, tonometer, eye speculum, eye forceps, corneal scissor, strabismus scissor, iris hook, air injection canula etc.

Figure 1.1 Surgical Instruments is given below

a.	Straight artery forceps	f.	Curved scissor
b.	Curved artery forceps	g.	Straight scissor
c.	Allis tissue forceps	h.	Rat tooth forceps
d.	Needle holder	i.	Towel clamp
e.	B. P handle and blade	j.	Different suture needle

Figure 1.2 Teat Instruments is given below

a.	Udder infusion tube	e.	Teat dilator
b.	Teat tumour extractor	f.	Teat siphon
c.	Teat slitter	g.	Teat scissor
d.	Teat bistoury	h.	Litchy teat knife

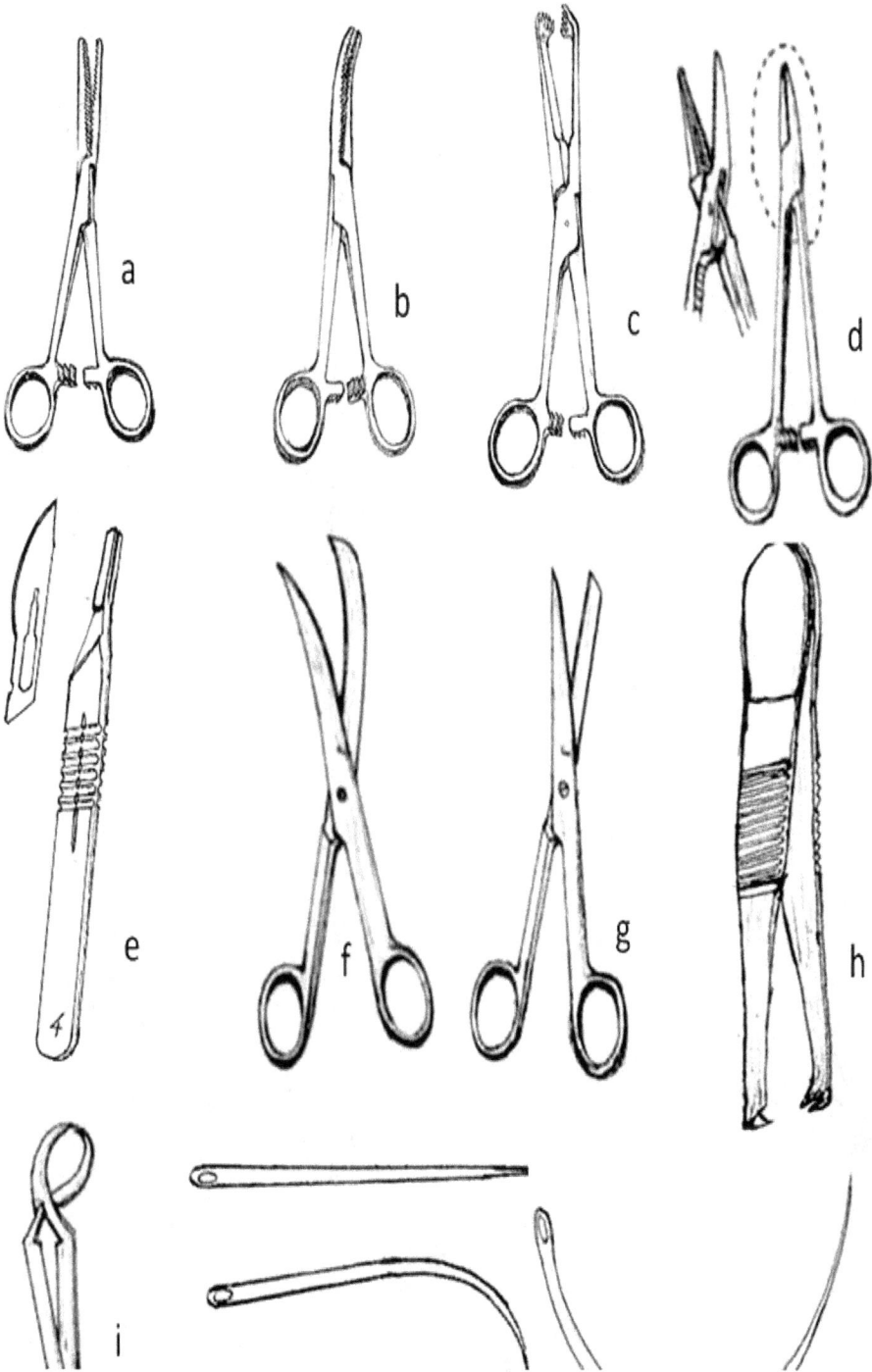

Figure 1.1 : Surgical Instruments

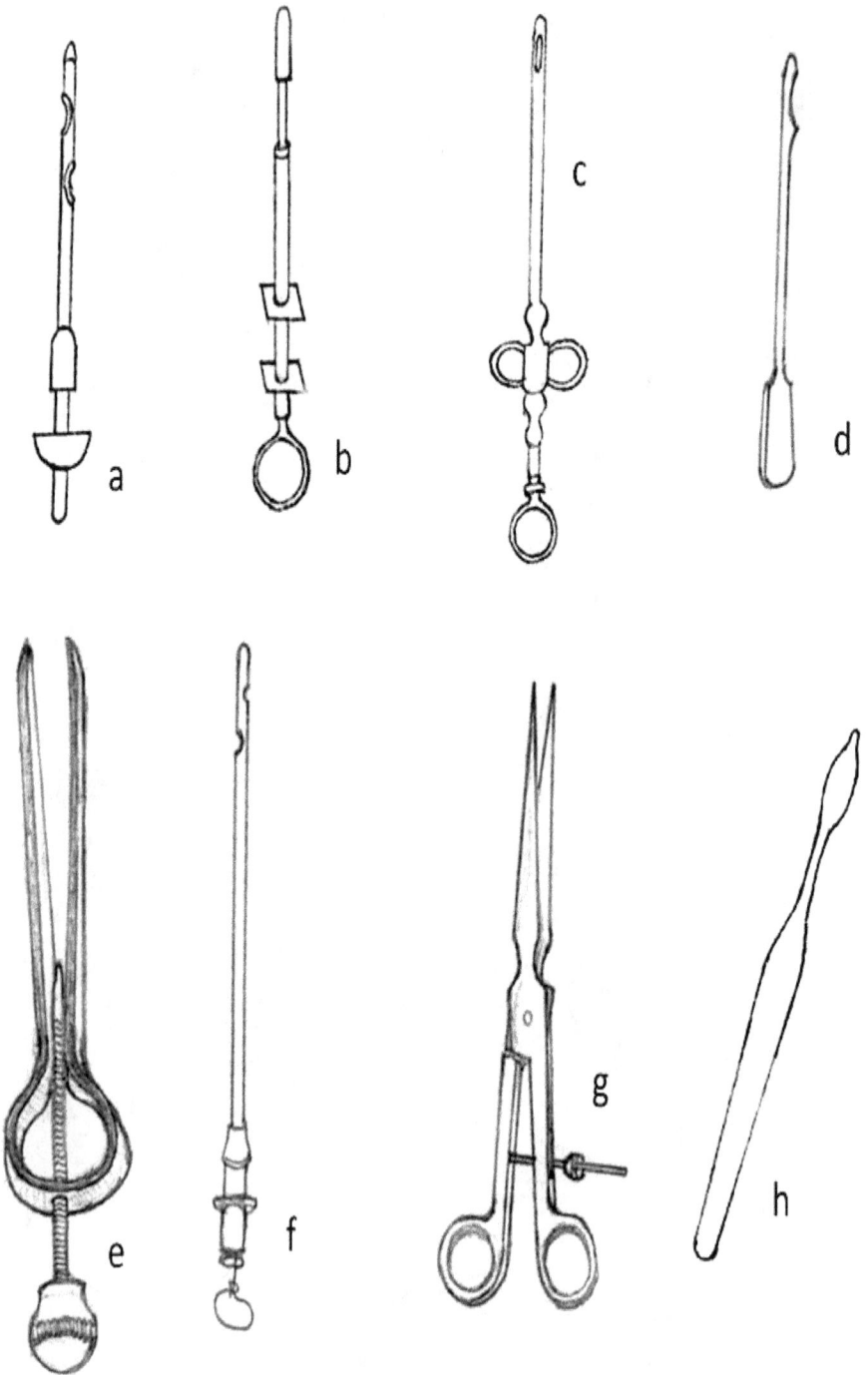

Figure 1.2: Teat Instruments

Chapter 2

Layout of Operation Theatre

A variety of physical layouts are suitable for modern operation theatre and surgical areas. The goal of all designs is patient safety and work efficiency. The surgical area should be located close to anaesthesia and surgical preparation areas, critical care, radiology and central supply. However, it should be isolated from general traffic flow (*i.e.* examination rooms, office, reception area, wards).

An ideal operation theatre consist of operation room, intensive care room, accident/emergency room, X-ray unit, laboratory unit and sterilization room grouped together to provide maximum use of equipments and skilled personnel. It should be so located that it is indecent of general traffic with separate disposal corridors. The entrance to the operating and personnel should have separate entry and exit points to ensure sterility. The clean zone consists of the scrub and gowning room and anaesthetic room. The clean zone should have adequate storage room for equipments, general supplies, sterile packs, X- ray and dark room with an adjacent, centralized sterilization and disinfecting unit.

Movement of personnel should be from one clean area to another. Sufficient ventilation must be provided in such a way that the airflow is from clean to less clean areas. All surfaces should be washable and the joints between walls and ceiling curved to minimize collection of dust.

In general the facilities and elementary features with adequate ventilation must be taken care off. The walls should be smooth, washable and should be withstand repeated application of detergents. Tiles are not advisable. The finish should be semi- matt so as to reduce infection. The colours of choice are pale blue, gray or green.

Lighting in the operating department is entirely dependent on artificial lighting with sufficient emergency backup. Ventilation must be such a way that

i.   It supplies heated or cooled, humidified, contamination free air to the operating area.

ii. It introduces air into these rooms to remove the contaminants liberated within.

iii. It prevents entry of air from contaminated areas.

Sections of Operation Theatre

1. Dressing room

Dressing rooms are used by surgeons to change into proper surgical suite. The dressing room should have closed cabinets for surgical scrub suits, shoe cover, masks and caps and a separate area for hanging street cloths. A hamper for dirty laundry should be available to minimize carrying contaminated linen throughout the hospital.

2. Anaesthesia and surgical preparation room

The surgical preparation and anaesthesia room should be located adjacent to the surgical area. This area should be supplied with equipment or medications that may be necessary in the event of an emergency. Anaesthetic equipments, laryngoscope, clippers, skin preparation materials, needles and syringes and monitoring equipment should be readily available to ensure efficient anaesthesia and preoperative patient preparation.

Stainless steel tables with inbuilt sinks are ideal for patient preparation. General lighting is achieved by main overhead fluorescent lights, supplemented by a spotlight directed at each preparation table.

3. Sterile instrument room

The sterile instruments room is a clean area in which all sterilized and packaged instruments and supplies.

4. Equipment room

Large equipment such as anaesthetic machines, lasers, monitoring equipment, operating microscopes and portable surgical lights can be stored in equipment room.

5. Scrub sink area

It should be located to the operating room suites. Antiseptic soap in an appropriate dispenser, scrub brushes and fingernail cleaners should be located within easy reach at each scrubbing station. Deep stainless steel sinks equipped with elbow or foot operated water activators are ideal.

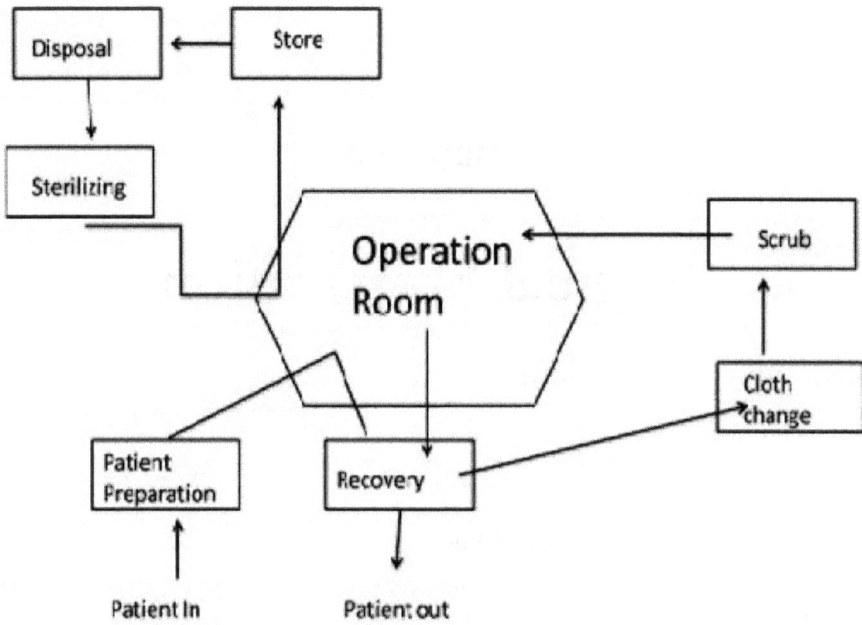

Figure 2.1: Traffic flows in an operating theatre

Chapter 3

Surgical Preparation

Preparation of General Surgical Pack

A general surgical pack is a sterilized bundle consisting of the usual surgical instruments, drapes, etc. required for the most of the common surgical operations.

A towel 36" x 36" size which will form the covering of the bundle. A 15" x 15" cloth is place over to keep the following instruments.

	Instrument	Quantity
i.	Suture materials	Sufficient quantity
ii.	Wound retractors	1 Pair
iii.	Suture needle	Different sizes
iv.	BP Handle No. 3	1 Nos.
v.	BP Handle No. 4	1 Nos.
vi.	Scissors (Straight and Curved)	1 Nos. Each
vii.	Towel clamp	8 Nos.
viii.	Artery forceps – straight	4 Nos.
ix.	Artery forceps – curved	4 Nos.
x.	Allies tissue forceps	4 Nos.
xi.	Rat tooth forceps	1 Nos.
xii.	Thumb forceps	1 Nos.
xiii.	Needle holder	1 Nos.
xiv.	Drape (Small animal)	1 Nos.
xv.	Drape (Large animal)	1 Nos.
xvi.	Gowns	1 Nos.
xvii.	Hand towels	2 Nos.
xviii.	Gauze pieces	Sufficient quantity

The bundle is made tight so as to lessen the quantity of air in it. This bundle is sterilized in the autoclave. Caps, masks and gloves are sterilized in a separate bundle.

Wrapping of Instrument Pack

- Wrap the instrument pack in a clean towel. Place large unfold wrap in front of you and position the instrument tray in the centre of the wrap.

- Fold the corner of the wrap that is closest to you over the instrument tray and to its far edges. Fold the tip of the wrap over so that it is exposed for easy unwrapping.

- Fold the right corner over the pack then, fold the left corner similarly.

- Turn the pack around and fold the final corner of the wrap over the tray, tucking it tightly under the previous two folds.

- Wrap the pack in a second layer of cloth or paper in a similar manner.

- Secure the last corner of the outer wrap with masking tape and a piece of heat sensitive indicator tape.

Preparation of Operative Site

The surgical site is prepared by shaving or clipping of the hairs from operative areas and some surrounding area. The shaved operative site is washed three or four time with soap and plenty of water till the dust, dirt is removed. Then site is scrubbed three or four times with antimicrobial agents. The site is cleaned with sterile cotton after each and every scrubbed. Precaution should be taken during cleaning of the operative site which is not affected by used cotton from one site to other. Cleaning should be start from line of incision and goes its periphery. The site should be making aseptic by use of 70 per cent isopropyl or ethyl alcohol and transfer the patient in operation room. The animal is anaesthestised by suitable anaesthetic agents and makes animal position as suitable for surgeon. Operative site should be cover by using of surgical drape, which help to maintain aseptic area.

Surgical Team

All personnel entering the operation theatre regardless of whether a surgery is in progress or not, should be appropriately clothed. They should wear scrub clothes rather than street clothes to minimize the microbial contamination. The sleeves of the top should be short enough to allow the hands and arms to be scrubbed. Also wear cap to cover the head and mask to cover the mouth and nostrils. Any footwear that is comfortable can be worn in the operation theatre. Shoe cover should be donned when first entering in the surgical area.

Scrubbing

Objectives of surgical scrub include mechanical removal of dirt and oil, reduction of the transient bacterial population and depression of the skins residual bacterial population. Before scrubbing all jewellery (including watches) should be removed from the hands and forearms because they are reservoir of bacteria. Fingernails should be free of polish and trimmed short and cuticles should be in good condition. Surgical scrubs are used to clean the hands and forearms to reduce bacterial numbers that come in contact with the wound. All surgical team members should scrub hand and arm before entering in the surgical suite. Commonly available surgical scrubs are chlorhexidine gluconate, hexachlorophene, iodophors, parachloromethaxylenol and triclosan.

Surgical scrub procedure

 - ➢ Locate scrub brushes, antimicrobial soap and nail cleaners.
 - ➢ Remove watch and rings.
 - ➢ Wet hands and forearms thoroughly.
 - ➢ Apply 2-3 pumps of antimicrobial soap to the hands and wash hands and forearms.
 - ➢ Clean nails and subungual areas with a nail cleaner under running water.
 - ➢ Rinse arms and forearms.
 - ➢ Apply 2-3 pumps of antimicrobial soap to hands and forearms.
 - ➢ Apply 2-3 pumps of antimicrobial soap to sterile scrub brushes.
 - ➢ Rinse the scrub brush well under running water and transfer the brush to your scrubbed hand. Do not rinse the scrubbed hand and arm at this time.
 - ➢ When both hand and arms have been scrubbed, drop the scrub in the sink.
 - ➢ Starting with the fingertips of one hand, rinse under water by moving your fingertips up and out of the water stream and allowing the rest of your arm to be rinsed off on the way out of the stream.
 - ➢ Always allow the water to run from your fingertips to elbows.
 - ➢ Never allow your fingertips to come below the level of your elbow.
 - ➢ Never shake your hands to get rid of excess water.
 - ➢ Hold your hands upright and in front of you so that they can be seen and proceed to the gowning and gloving area.

Gowning

It should be done from a surface separate from other sterile supplies or the surgical patient to avoid dripping water on the sterile field and contaminating it. Grasp the gown firmly and gently lifts it away from the table. Hold the gown at shoulder and allow it to gently unfold. Once gown is opened identify the armholes and guide each arm through the sleeves. Keep hands within the cuffs of the gown. An assistant to pull the gown up over your shoulders and secure it by closing the neck fasteners and tie inside the wrist.

Gloving

Pick up on glove by its inner cuff with the opposite hand. Slide the glove on to the opposite hand; leave the cuff down. Using the partially glove hand, slide your fingers into the outer side of the opposite glove cuff. Slide your hand into the glove and unfold the cuff.

Sterilization

Sterilization is a process by which an article can be rendered free from all forms of living microbes including bacteria, fungi and their spores, and viruses. On the basis of the magnitude of the risk of infection involved in the use of the material, the surgical instruments and equipments can be classified into three categories.

1. When the risk is great, items are critical. Most of these items are introduced beneath the surface of patients' body *e.g.,* surgical pack instruments.

2. The semi critical items like endotracheal tubes come in direct contact with mucous membranes but the body has barrier to infection.

3. The non-critical items are those, which do not make a direct contact with the patient. *e.g.,* face masks and rebreathing bag. It is not always necessary to use sterile semi critical and non-critical items; however, these must be clean and not contaminated.

Sterilization can be achieved by three methods: heat, chemical and radiation.

Heat

Sterilization by heat is the oldest and most widely used and recognized process. Moist heat is more effective than dry heat and requires lower temperature and lesser time. Articles must be cleaned thoroughly before sterilization. Spores show maximum resistance to heat at neutral pH and so increased acidity or alkalinity decrease this resistance. For this reason two per cent sodium carbonate (washing soda) is added to water used for sterilization by boiling. Sodium carbonate also slightly raises the boiling point of water and reduces blunting and rusting of the instruments. Heat sterilization involves either dry or moist heat. The methods of dry heat sterilization include direct exposure of instruments to flame and the use of a hot air oven. The flame method is not reliable and so hot air ovens are used. Dry heat destroys microbes primarily by oxidation process. It is used to sterilize those materials for which moist heat cannot be used either due to deleterious effects on the material or material being impermeable to steam *e.g.,* oils, powder, sealed containers etc. Sterilization by dry heat is a slow process and long exposure time at a high temperature is required as spores are relatively resistant to dry heat.

Various temperature and time combinations given for dry heat sterilization are 120 C for 8 hours, 140 C for 60 minutes and 170 C for 40 minutes. Exposure times related to the time after specific temperature has been achieved and do not include heating lags. Selection of temperature shall depend upon the resistance of the material to the heat. Clean gowns, drapes and paper wrapped material (swabs, petri dishes etc.) can be sterilized at 120 C in 8 hours. Higher temperature will burn the paper and fabric. Stainless steel items and glassware can be sterilized at 160 C in 60 minutes. Materials, which can be sterilized by dry heat in an oven, include glassware, glass syringes, dry material in sealed containers, powders, oils, swabs, drapes etc.

Moist heat in the form of saturated steam under pressure is the most dependable and recognized method of sterilization. A variety of autoclaves are available for the purpose, which use steam under pressure. In routine, materials are autoclaved at 121 C under 15 lbs pressures for 30 minutes. The procedure provides moisture and heat under pressure, which is more effective than dry heat. Sharp instruments like scissors, needles and other routine instruments of a surgical pack, excluding sharp scalpel blades, can be autoclaved without reducing their life.

Moist heat sterilization includes boiling in water and use of an autoclave. Boiling of instruments in water at 100 C for 10-15 minutes can be used in an emergency as a lesser method of sterilization.

Proper loading and correct packing are the prerequisites for effective sterilization by autoclaving. An autoclave is ineffective if the items are tightly packed and the steam fails to penetrate all items. While preparing the pack, the locks and joints of the instruments should be kept open and the complex instruments, like orthopaedic equipment, should be dissembled. Once the material has been sterilized, it should be wrapped in paper to avoid penetration of dust and dirt, if items are not to be used immediately. If an autoclaved pack is wrapped in a double layer of muslin cloth, it remains sterilized on open shelves for three weeks and in closed cabinets for seven week; Sterilization of the pack can be monitored by incorporating test indicator strips, one each inside and outside the pack. Under field conditions, if an autoclave is not available, a large capacity pressure cooker can be used to sterilize a surgical pack. In these conditions, pressure should be maintained for 45 minutes and test indicator labels should be used to be on safer side.

Chemical

Chemical or cold sterilization is often used for sharp edged instruments, like scalpel blades and hypodermic needles. Absolute ethyl alcohol or one per cent cetrimide can be used for continuous immersion of the needles for ready use. It is recommended that sodium nitrite (4 g/L) should be added to the sterilizing solution to prevent rusting of the instruments. Some surgeons also use chemicals to sterilize surgical instruments in an emergency or when an autoclave is not available. Commercially prepared solutions like Cidex and Sterisol are available for this purpose. Exposure time varies from a few to 24 hours depending upon the solution used. Such preparations mostly contain two per cent gluteraldehyde or one to two per cent formaldehyde. With the later solution, up to 24 hours are required to kill the spores and prolonged aeration is necessary. Due to irritant nature of the solutions, instruments must be rinsed in saline before use. Instruments can also be disinfected by two minutes immersion in 1:30 concentration of Savlon in 70 per cent ethyl alcohol. However, chemical sterilization is not a substitute to autoclaving but can be used suitably for disinfections of endotracheal tubes, plastic sheets and drainage catheters. Sterilization by using ethylene oxide can be considered as an alternative to autoclaving but is expensive.

Ethyl alcohol and isopropyl alcohol are effective antiseptics with persistent antibacterial effect. A 70 per cent ethyl or isopropyl alcohol had maximum germicidal action because of presence of water that easily denatures the protein. A 70 per cent alcohol is more germicidal than absolute alcohol. Isopropyl alcohol is more bactericidal than ethyl alcohol. Bulky rubber goods, gumboots etc., can be disinfected with a solution containing 135 ml of formalin (38 per cent) and 10 g of sodium hydroxide in one litre of distilled water. Material should remain immersed in the solution for at least two hours.

Radiation

Non-ionising radiation, *e.g.*, from Ultraviolet lamps, is generated by a special source of mercury vapour commonly known as germicidal lamp. Ultraviolet radiation from the lamp can be used to sterilize operation theatre. Ionising radiations includes X-rays and gamma rays and are very lethal to living cells. Such radiation is used to sterilize packed items like disposable syringes, catheters, endotracheal tubes, intravenous sets etc.

Chapter 4

Suture

Sutures or surgical threads have been employed since ancient times. They are used to hold the cut edges of tissues in close approximation during healing to hold implants and to ligate blood vessels for prompt haemostasis.

Ideal suture material should possess and maintain adequate tensile strength till healing is achieved; be non capillary, non carcinogenic, non allergic and non electrolytic. It should be easy to handle, maintain a knot without tendency to slip, loosen or swell due to wetting, incite minimum tissue reaction and be inexpensive. The material should be readily available and easily sterilized without much alteration in its tensile strength and other physical and chemical characteristics.

The degree of tensile strength of a suture materials determines whether the material is absorbable or non absorbable. Absorbable suture material is bio-degraded and eliminated from the body within 60 days through phagocytosis by macrophage. Such materials are used for short term immobilization of wound edges e.g. suturing of viscera, peritoneum, muscle etc. Non-absorbable material resists biodegradation and retains its tensile strength for more than 60 days and thereby necessitates its removal. When used in internal organs/structure, fibrous tissue encapsulates non- absorbable materials. Such material is require where long-term immobilization of tissue or parts is necessary e.g. retention of prosthesis or when tissue apposed are subjected to movement and heal slowly e.g. tendon, ligament and bone. Suture material may be prepared from natural fibers, metals or synthetic polymers. A suture may be monofilament or multifilament, the later may be braided.

Absorbable Suture Material

Catgut

Catgut is the most widely used absorbable materials in veterinary surgery. It is obtained either from the submucosa of the ovine small intestine or the serosal layer of the bovine small intestine. It is composed of formaldehyde treated collagen fibres and multifilament material having capillary action. It can be sterilized by ionizing radiation or by ethylene oxide; however, the latter prolongs its absorption time. Catgut is available in presterilised aluminium foils containing 85 per cent ethyl alcohol. It cannot be autoclaves as heat denatures the protein and hence the tensile strength of the material is reduced.

Catgut is available in plain or chromatized form. Catgut is treated with chromic acid solution to increased its tensile strength and absorption time and decrease the tissue reaction, catgut is categorized depending on the degree of chromatization; type A (plain), type B (mild chromic), type C (medium chromic) and type D (extra chromic) and loss of tensile strength takes 5,10,20 and 40 days, respectively. The material is available in sizes varying from No. 7/0 (finest) to No. 3 (thickest).The normal length of available catgut is 152 cm. Depending on the thickness the catgut is numbered as under.

Size (thickness in mm)	Size No.
1.016	7
0.914	6
0.813	5
0.711	4} Used for suturing hernia ring, fascia etc. in large
0.635	3} animals.
0.559	2} Muscle suture and suturing of organ in large
0.483	1} animals.
0.406	0 (1/0)} Used for bowel suture and ligation of Vessels.
0.330	00(2/0)}
0.254	000 (3/0) Eye surgery
0.203	0000 (4/0)

General size recommended for specific tissues are as under.

- ❖ Ligation of large vessels and pedicles : (0 to 2/0)
- ❖ Fascia and dense connective tissue in small animals : (0 to 3/0)
- ❖ Fascia and dense connective tissue in large animals : (0 to 2)
- ❖ Skin and subcutaneous tissue : (0 to 4/0)
- ❖ The skin graft and small vessels : (3/0 to 4/0)
- ❖ Gastrointestinal and urogenital surgery : (3/0 to 4/0)
- ❖ Vascular surgery : (3/0 to 6/0)
- ❖ Nerve sheaths : (5/0 to 4/0)

As plain catgut incites severe tissue reaction and rapidly losses its strength, it is not used routinely in surgery. In routine surgical procedures, mild to medium chronic catgut is used. It is absorbed and digested by macrophages and lysosomal enzymes. Although relatively easy to handle, catgut weakens and swells in vivo and hence results in poor knots getting united.

Collagen

Collagen is a multifilament suture material obtained from bovine flexor tendon and treated with formaldehyde or chromic acid or both. It incites less tissue reaction than catgut but absorption is similar. Fine collagen is used in ophthalmic surgery.

Kangaroo tendon

It is harvested from the Kangaroo. It has high tensile strength, so it can be used in slow healing tissue or where greater strength of the suture material is require, such as in joint capsule or for hernia repair.

Facia lata

Facia lata is obtained from bovine. It can be use to provide additional support to fascial layers.

Polyglycolic acid

It is soft and flexible, stimulates less tissue reaction and is completely absorbed in 100 to 200 days. It is synthetic, noncollagen, braided multifilament, polymer glycolic acid. It is absorbed by hydrolysis and digestion. The material has greater tensile strength than catgut but loss of strength is more rapid making it unsuitable for use in slow healing tissue. It is available in sizes from numbers six zero to two.

Polyglactin 910

It is a synthetic, monofilament braided suture material. It is sterilized by ethylene oxide and may be coated or uncoated, hydrolysis and absorption occurs in 40 to 90 days. The suture has an excellent size to strength ratio, relatively easy to handle, stable in contaminated wound and elicit minimum tissue reaction. This suture material is used in teat surgery, abdominal surgery and ophthalmic surgery routinely.

Polydioxanone (PDS)

Polydioxanone is more flexible than polyglycolic acid and polyglactine 910. It is a synthetic, monofilament polymer of paradioxanone. It is sterilized by ethylene oxide. It incites little tissue reaction.

Non absorbable materials

Silk

It is inexpensive, readily available and easily sterilized by autoclaving. It is obtained from cocoon of silkworm, processed to remove its natural waxes and gums, and dyed with a vegetable dye. The main disadvantage is the high degree of tissue reaction. The material binds with gamma globulins, which eventually leads to acute inflammation. The material should not be used to close contaminated wound, as the fibres will hold blood that is an excellent medium for bacterial proliferation.

Cotton

Cotton is inexpensive and readily available. Its tensile strength and knot security is more when wet. It causes slightly less tissue reaction than silk. Disadvantages include capillary tissue reaction and ability to potentiate infection.

Umbilical tape

Umbilical tape suture is mostly used to tie the umbilical cord of the newborn or as vulvar sutures in case of prolapse of the vagina or uterus. It is also used to close the defect following abdominal hernia.

Linen

Surgical linen is a braided material obtained from vegetable fibres. It has less tensile strength but relatively good knot security.

Stainless steel

Stainless steel suture is available as simple or twisted. It can be easily sterilized by autoclaving and incites no inflammatory reaction as it is a completely bio-inert material. It has the highest tensile strength and greatest knot security among all the suture materials available. It is used to hold slow healing tissues like ligaments, tendons and bones. Simple stainless steel sutures can be used in contaminated and infected wounds. The main disadvantage of stainless steel is its poor handling quality. Moreover, it has tendency to cut through the tissues and may break down following repeated bending.

Nylon

It is biologically inert and may be monofilament or multifilament, the former is noncapillary. Nylon stimulates minimal tissue reaction. Monofilament nylon can be used for closing cutaneous wounds. It has poor handling characteristics and knot security.

Vetafil

This is a non-irritant, noncapillary synthetic fibre. Sizes commonly used are medium, extra heavy and special.

Polypropylene

Polypropylene is inert, incites minimal tissue reaction, but it is slippery and not very easy to handle. It is a monofilament polymer of propylene. It has low tensile strength but high knot strength. It is sterilized by ethylene oxide. It can be used on the skin, cardiac muscle and infected wounds due to high flexibility.

Table 4.1: Commonly available suture material

Sr. No	Name of the suture material	Trade name	Suture character- istic	Absorp- tion (days)	Tissue reaction
1	Catgut	Catgut	Absorbable multi-filament	60	+++
2	Polyglactin 910	Vicryl	Absorbable multi-filament	60	+
3	Polyglycolic acid	Dexon	Absorbable multi-filament	60-90	+
4	Polydiaoxanone	PDS II	Absorbable multi-filament	180	+
5	Polyglyconate	Maxon	Absorbable multi-filament	180	+
6	Silk	Perma hand	Non-absorbable multifilament	> 2 years	+++
7	Polyester	Mersiline Ethi-bond	Non-absorbable multifilament		++
8	Polyamide (Nylon)	Ethilon Nurolon	Non-absorbable monofilament Multifilament		
9	Polypropylene	Prolene	Non-absorbable monofilament		-
10	Polybutester	Novafil	Non-absorbable monofilament		-
11	Stainless steel	Flexon	Non-absorbable monofilament Multifilament		-

Suture Techniques

Interrupted sutures

These sutures are employed mostly for approximation of the skin edges. Apart from, this they are also employed for approximation of the linea alba in small animals, lower abdominal wall, hernial ring etc. Since every suture is independent holding power is better. Further, it bears a thin faint scar after healing. In this the threaded needle is passed from outside inside of one edge and taken out inside outside from the other edge and surgical knot is tied. The distance between two sutures is approximately about 2 cm. The tension over the sutures should only be so much so as to oppose the skin edges.

Simple continuous sutures

These sutures are employed for approximation of peritoneum, fascia, cut in thin muscles, etc. Since the sutures are continuous and knotting is done only in the beginning and end of the sutures, if the knot gets loosened whole approximation gets disrupted. Hence the holding strength is not sufficient and as such this type of suture is not employed wherever there is tension over the edges. However, the method is quick. First the threaded needle is passed from out-side inside of one edge and taken out from inside out-side from the other edge. A surgical knot is tied. Without cutting the thread the suturing is continued in the same pattern without knotting till whole the cut edge is approximated and the surgical knot is tied.

Continuous lock stitch sutures

These sutures are also known as blanket sutures or Cobler's sutures. It is employed for approximating hernial ring during diaphragmatic hernia operation. The sutures have the same advantages and disadvantages of simple continuous sutures. However, they are firmer. The technique is started as simple continuous suture but after completion of the next bite the threaded needle is taken below the thread of the previous suture. This pattern continued till the approximation is complete. The ending of the suture is similar to that of simple continuous suture.

Mattress sutures

There are two types of mattress sutures.

i.   Horizontal mattress sutures

ii. Vertical mattress sutures

Since these are interrupted type of sutures and each involves more amount of tissue, they have a good holding capacity. The method also helps in obliterating the underlying dead space.

In horizontal mattress sutures the threaded needle is passed from outside inside (1st bite) about 1 cm away from one edge and is taken out (2nd bite) at the same distance from the other edge. Now the needle (3rd bite) is taken outside inside about 2 cm away but parallel to the wound edge of the same side. Then the threaded needle is taken out (4th bite) again about first cm away from the skin edge of the other side. The free ends of thread are knotted. Thus the distance of all the 4 bites from the wound edge is about 1 cm and that off stand 4th and 2nd and 3rd is about 2 cm. The next suture is started about 2 cm away from the 1 suture and suturing in this manner is continued till the wound edges are completely approximated. This will result in aversion of would edges and because of this it will leave a thick distinct scar after healing.

The principle of vertical mattress suture is same. However in this technique all the four needle points will come in the same line and perpendicular to the wound edges. These sutures are stronger than the horizontal sutures.

Lembert suture

These sutures are employed on the hollow organs having serous layer. The principle is to approximate serous layers on completion of the suturing. The serous layers, when apposed, deposit fibrin and the wound gets sealed within few days. In this type of suture the mucous membrane is not included in the suture. The needle bite (1st bite) is taken about 2 to 3 mm away from the wound edge and taken out (2nd bite) about 1 to 2 mm away from the wound edge of the same side without penetrating the mucous membrane. Then the needle is pierced (3rd bite) about 1 to 2 mm away from the wound edge of the other side and is taken out (4th bite) about 2 to 3 mm away from the same wound edge again without piercing the mucous membrane. A surgical knot is tied and similar type of suturing is continued in a continuous pattern till the wound edges are closed. This results into inversion of the wound edges opposing the serous layers. The sutures line is perpendicular to the wound edge. Too much of tissue should not be included in the bite, especially while suturing the intestines to avoid diaphragm formation. It is advisable to rephrase the first suture line with another layer of Lembert sutures. Atraumatic needle should be used for suturing.

Czerny sutures

This pattern is almost same as Lembert suture. But the 2nd bite is at the edge of the wound *i.e.* the needle is taken out at the edge just above the mucous membrane. Likewise for the 3rd bite the needle is pierced from the sub mucous layer. The only advantage with this method is that it involves less amount of tissue. However, another layer of Lembert sutures must reinforce it.

Cushing suture

This pattern is also similar to Lembert sutures except that the suture bite is parallel to the wound edge without involving the mucous membrane. When compared to Lembert sutures there are two advantages with this method.

(i) It involves less amount of tissue in the suture bite, thus diaphragm formation is avoided.

(ii) Since the suture line is parallel to the wound edge the union is stronger.

For this pattern of suturing round-bodied needle should be used.

Connell suture

These sutures are similar to cushing sutures except that the mucous membrane is also included in the suture's bite. It is employed for approximation of intestines and sometimes urinary bladder also. Reinforcement of the suture line with a layer of cushing or Lembert's suture is a must when this method is employed.

Overlapping sutures

This is a special type of suture technique employed for the closure of the hernial ring. The pattern is just like horizontal mattress sutures. However mode of passing the needle differs. The first needle bite is taken from outside inside from one edge of the ring and taken out from the other edge again outside inside. The third and the 4th bites are taken inside outside and the free ends of the thread are knotted. This results into overlapping of the first edge over the second edge.

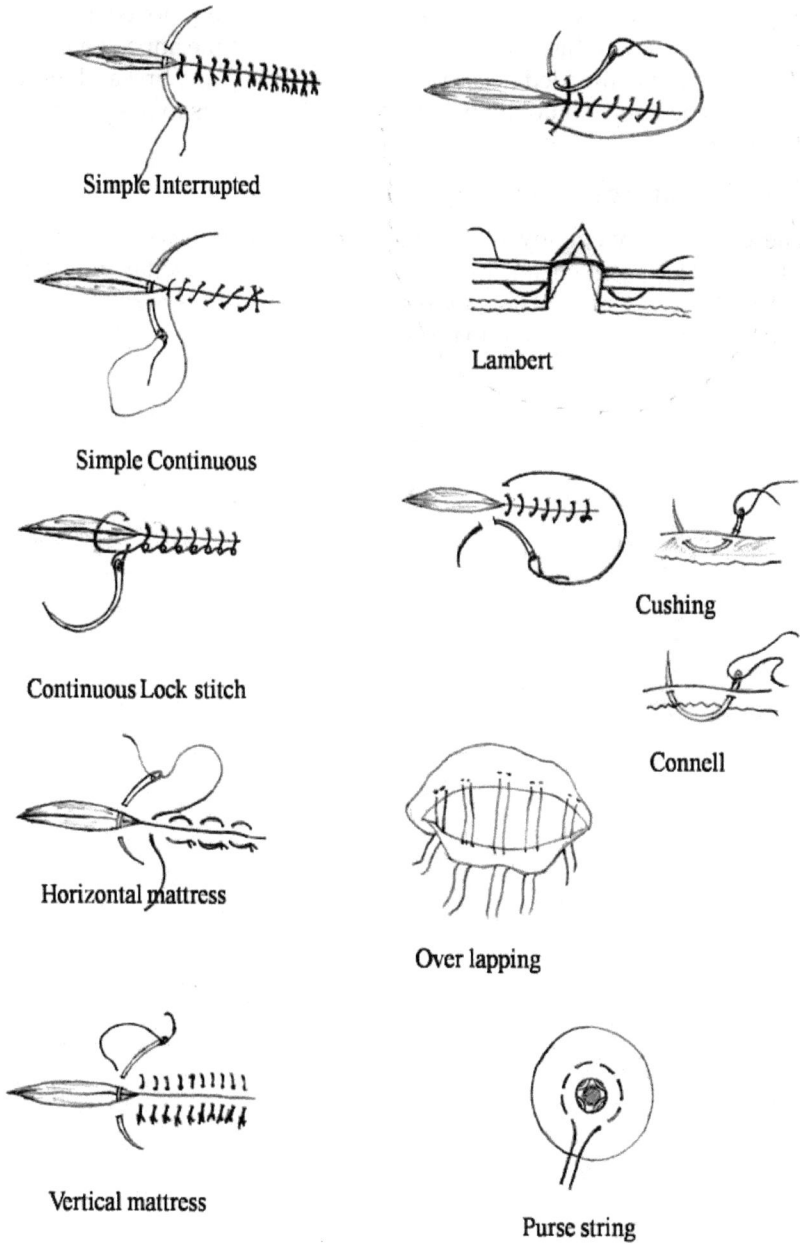

Figure 4.1: Suture technique

Purse string suture

It is also known as tobacco pouch sutures. It is employed for temporary closure of anal ring. In this, folds of the skin all around the anus at equal distance are pierced with the threaded needle and the free ends of the first and the last folds are knotted. The knot should not be too tight. A space so as to pass a finger should be there for the feces to void.

Relaxation sutures or tension sutures

These sutures are employed to relax the tension over the primary closure. The threaded needle is passed far away from wound edge and taken out again far away from the other edge. The knot is put on the free ends of the thread. Two or three such sutures are sufficient to relax tension over the primary closure.

Chapter 5

Haemostesis

The presence of blood during the course of an operation covers the field of surgery and its accumulation in the wound afterwards favors bacterial growth.

Technique to control haemorrhage

1. **Use of Tourniquet:** The tourniquet is applied in the form of a band or cord tightly round the limb or appendage above the seat of operation.

2. **Use of Esmarch's bandage:** Elastic bandage applied from the distal part of the extremity to a point above the seat of operation. Tourniquet is then applied and bandage is removed.

3. **Digital compression:** Pressure maintained on the chief vessel of supply by the fingers of an assistant.

4. **hypodermaly injection of Adrenaline:** Adrenaline can be injected hypodermaliy to prevent capillary haemorrhage.

5. **Thermocautery:** Dull heat leads to retraction of the coats of the blood vessels and contraction, resulting in diminished lumen and clot formation on the orifice.

6. **Crushing:** The ecraseur or artery forceps can be used to crush the vessels.

7. **Tearing:** Tearing of the tissue is often employed in the removal of tumors loosely attached and situated in the vicinity of the vessels.

8. **Blunt dissection:** Blunt dissection is performed by rupturing the tissues by a blunt instrument. This method is employed for the isolation of a large vessel like jugular vein and carotid artery.

9. **Ligation:** Legation of the bleeding vessels with silk or catgut. This is the surest method of arresting bleeding.

10. **Torsion:** Torsion is sufficient to arrest haemorrhage from smaller vessels. Bleeding end of the vessels is secured with artery forceps drawn out slightly and twisted on its long axis several times.

11. **Forcipressure:** Forcipressure consists of applying an artery forceps to the end of the vessel and leaving it in this position until it is convenient to apply ligature.

12. **Crushing of Arterioles:** Performed by special strong forceps.

13. **Plugging or Packing a hollow wound:** Packing the cavity with medicated gauze or cotton wool can prevent haemorrhage from the hollow wound.

14. **Application of styptics:** Adrenaline, astringent lotions, tincture benzoine, ice and cold water can be applied to minimize bleeding.

Chapter 6

Inhalation Anaesthesia

Inhalation anaesthesia is relatively safe because the effect can be reversed. The use of inhalation anaesthesia is comparatively expansive and require inhalation equipments. Different methods of inhalation anaesthesia are as under.

Open drop method

In the past inhalation anaesthetics agents were soaked in sponges or to towels and placed in masks around the patient's mouth. Open systems have no-reservoir and do not allow for rebreathing e.g., Ether and Chloroform. Disadvantages are neither control over anaesthetic concentration nor control of patient's respiratory function.

Closed method

Closed system has a reservoir and allows for complete rebreathing of all exhaled gases except CO_2, which is taken up by CO_2 absorber. CO_2 is removed by conversion into calcium hydroxide.

Semi closed non rebreathing circuits

Principal of semi closed non rebreathing circuits is fresh gases flow from the anaesthetic machine into a reservoir, from which the patient inhales. The exhaled gases are spilled to atmosphere. In veterinary anaesthesia, commonly used semi closed non breathing circuits are the Magill circuit, 'T' piece circuit and axial circuit. The exhaled gases are directed into a closed bag and after CO_2 absorption, O_2 are added at higher flow rate and excess gases are allowed to escape through an overflow valve.

Different types of inhalation anaesthetics

Inhalant anaesthetic are available like Halothane, Isoflurane, Sevoflurane, Desflurane and Nitrous oxide. The advantages are patent airway, rapid control of anaesthetic depth, quick and smooth recovery, and disadvantages are more pronounced cardiovascular depression including myocardial depression, hypotension and bradycardia.

1. Nitrous oxide

Analgesia from N_2O reduces inhalational anaesthetic requirement therefore less cardiovascular depression. However, the potency of nitrous oxide is only half that of human, so the sparing effect is not as obvious. Use of this agent is not widespread in dogs.

2. Isoflurane

Used to be much more expensive than halothane, but now much more affordable and has replaced halothane both in human and veterinary markets worldwide. Quicker anaesthetic stabilization and more rapid recovery than halothane due to its lower blood gas solubility. Vapor setting is at 3-4 per cent in dogs at induction with oxygen flow at 60 ml/kg/min and is reduced between 1.5-3 per cent during the maintenance with oxygen flow at 20 ml/kg/min. Isoflurane, similar to halothane, induces a dose-dependent cardiovascular depression. Isoflurane causes more peripheral vasodilatation than halothane, which is responsible for a low arterial blood pressure, but tissue looks more bright and pinky indicating better perfusion. Isoflurane is less prone to cause arrhythmia compared to halothane

3. Sevoflurane

Anaesthetic induction, recovery, and intraoperative modulation of anaesthetic depths to be notably faster than halothane and Isoflurane. More expensive than halothane and isoflurane, but it is getting less expensive. Sevoflurane (1 MAC = 2.3 per cent) is less potent than halothane or Isoflurane, but more potent than desflurane. Sevoflurane induces dose dependent cardiovascular depression to a degree similar to that of isoflurane.

4. Desflurane

It has lower blood/gas partition coefficient than the other inhalants like Nitrous oxide, isoflurane, Sevoflurane, so control of anaesthetic depth is the quick among the volatile agents in clinical use. The least potent among the volatile anaesthetics (MAC = 8~11 per cent). Cardiovascular effects of desflurane are similar with those of Isoflurane. Expensive as sevoflurane and requires electronically controlled vaporizer which adds to the inconvenience

5. Halothane

MAC of halothane in dog is 0.8 per cent. Vapor setting is at 3-4 per cent at induction with oxygen flow at 60 ml/kg/min and is reduced between 1-3 per cent during the maintenance with oxygen flow at 20 ml/kg/min. As anaesthesia is deepened by increasing halothane concentration, CO_2 and arterial pressure decrease further. Heart rate is usually remains constant.

Inhalant anaesthesia machine (Boyels apparatus)

Anaesthesia machine use to prepare precise and safe mixture of anaesthetics gas and carrier gas which supply to the breathing system. Various anaesthesia machine are use to deliver this mixture to the patient but relatively sophisticated, precise, expensive instrument are use to deliver the volatile anaesthetics to the patient. Most anaesthetic delivery systems contain the same components. They reduce the high pressure of compressed gases and allow precise mixing with potent inhalant anaesthetics for safe delivery to the patient through breathing circuits. Primary components of machine which are necessary for the delivery of the volatile anaesthetics to the patient are describe in detail below.

An anaesthetic machine can be functionally subdivided into the following four components:

1. High pressure system.

    Where the pipeline and cylinder gas supplies are attached.

2. Low pressure system.

    Where O_2 and volatile anaesthetics are mixed.

3. Breathing system.

    Where the anaesthetic gas mixture is delivered to the patient.

4. Scavenging system.

Where excess gas from the breathing system is collected and diverted into the waste gas evacuation system.

Parts of anaesthetics machines

Various part of anaesthesia machine are as following and each part of machine have its own important.

1. Gas cylinder
2. Regulators and valves
3. Pressure gauges
4. Oxygen flush valve
5. Vaporizers

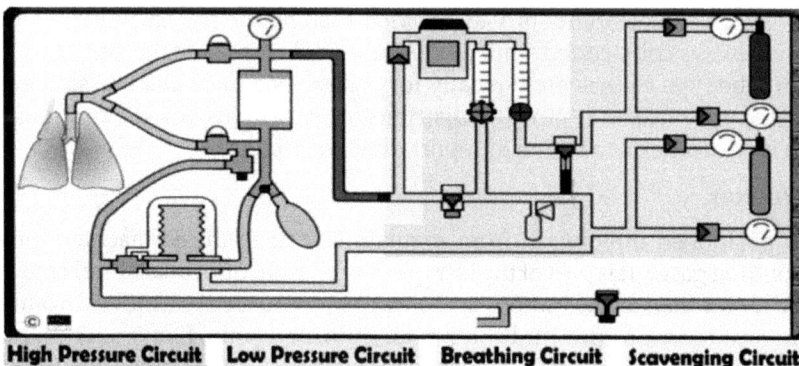

High Pressure Circuit   Low Pressure Circuit   Breathing Circuit   Scavenging Circuit

Figure 6.1: Diagram show function system of anaesthesia machine

1. Gas cylinders

Gas cylinder is the basic part of the anaesthesia machine which supplies the carrier gas and gaseous inhalation anaesthetics to the breathing circuit.

Table 6.1: Colour code of gas cylinders

Name of gases	Shoulder colour	Colour code
Oxygen	White	Black
Nitrous oxide	Blue	Blue
Carbon dioxide	Grey	Grey
Air	White / black quarter	Grey

2. Pressure regulator (Pressure reducing valves).

Pressure reducing valves are built into most anaesthetic machines. High-pressure gas within the cylinder is a danger to the patient and the pressure regulator reduces it to working level of 45 Psi. This ensures that high pressure gas does not enter to the flowmeter. It maintains constant flow in response to changes of pressure in a cylinder. It allows a wide range of flowmeter settings. The difference in pressure (pipeline gas at 50 Psi; cylinder gas at 45 Psi) forces the anaesthetic machine preferentially use gas supply from the pipe line gas when both sources are attached to the anaesthetic machine.

Function

- Safety relief (at 2 or 4 times the pressure in low pressure chamber)
- To protect equipment and personnel
- Prevent flowmeter fluctuations as cylinders empty
- Decrease sensitivity of flowmeter indicator to slight movement in control knob

3. Pressure gauges

Each compressed gas supplied to an anaesthesia machine should have corresponding pressure gauges. It is attach to the regulator for large cylinder and manifolds for bank of cylinders. Gauges identified by the gas chemical symbol or name and always color coded. Unit of measure is kilopascal on the gauges and Psi. Bourdon tube type gauges are typically for anaesthesia machine. Pressure gauges are also incorporated into pipeline distribution system at various locations. It is also use in anaesthesia machine to report pipeline pressure.

4. Flowmeter

It is positioned downward from regulators in anaesthesia machine for each corresponding gases. It is part of the low pressure system of an anaesthesia machine. The tube larger than at the bottom and a greater volume of gas moves around the indicator as it rises. Gas flow indicates in ml/min. or L/min. Flowmeter calibrated at 760 mm Hg and 20 °C, and accuracy may change under other conditions. A flowmeter's indicator should be read at the top except for ball-type float, which read at the center. The most common gas flowmeter is contains a ball or bobbin that rises within a glass tube to a height proportional to the flow of gas passing through the tube; the gas flow rate is read at the widest diameter of the ball or bobbin. A crack in the flowmeter may result in hypoxic mixture and the oxygen flowmeter should be the last in a series of flowmeter to avoid this.

Function

- Measure and indicate the rate of flow of gas, and enable precise control of O_2 and N_2O delivery to out of system vaporizers and to the common gas outlets.

- Flowmeter control the flow rate at which a specific gas passes through them.

5. Oxygen flush valve

It allows the gas bypass the vaporizer and delivers directly to the anaesthetic circuit via the common gas outlet. It delivers oxygen flow between 35 to 75 L/min. Beware as this large amount of gas delivery can over-pressurize small-sized lungs, particularly in a non-rebreathing circuit, resulting in a pneumothorax. It dilutes the anaesthetic concentration in the breathing circuit. It is best to fill the breathing circuit using flow control valve (flowmeter).

6. Vaporizers

Vaporizers are designed to change liquid anaesthetics into its vapors and add a specific amount of vapors to the gases being delivered to the patient. Saturated vapor pressure of anaesthetics is greater than partial pressure required for clinical anaesthesia (i.e. < MAC). So the design of precision vaporizers allows dilution of a high concentration of anaesthetic vapors from the vaporization chamber to a clinically usable and safe concentration. Heat is required for vaporization of liquid anaesthetics. Vaporizer made up of copper and bronze because of the favorable value of these metals for specific heat and thermal conductivity. More recently stainless steel has been used in construction of vaporizers.

7. Common gas outlet

It is exit from the anaesthetic machine for blended gas mixtures of carrier gas and volatile anaesthetics. Most machine outlets have a 15 mm inner diameter slip joint connection (that will accept a tracheal tube connector) with a 22 mm connection for outer diameter. It is a frequent source of gas leaks, so some machines come with a retaining device at the connection to make it harder to disengage.

Component of breathing system

Component of breathing system are the part of machine which are as following.

1. Fresh gas inlet

After passing through the vaporizer, the oxygen and inhalation anaesthetics enter in low pressure hose that delivers the fresh gas to the patient breathing circuit.

2. Rebreathing bag

Fresh gas entering the circuit is conveyed to an inflatable rubber reservoir bag. The bag is gradually filled as gases enter the circuit and is deflated with inhalation. The reservoir bag should have a minimum volume of 60 ml/kg of patient weight. The reservoir bag is easier for the patient to breathe from than a continuous flow of air. It also allows the anesthetist to deliver oxygen (with or without anaesthetic) by means of 'bagging'. The bag should be maintained partly full. It should not be allowed to overfill as this can cause serious lung damage by creating excessive pressure in the breathing circuit. If the reservoir bag is completely full either:

- The pop-off valve is closed.
- The patient is not breathing.
- The oxygen flow is set too high.
- The bag is too small.

The bag should not be completely deflated as this defeats its purpose as a reservoir. Complete emptying of the bag indicates that

- The gas flow is inadequate.
- The bag is too large.
- A leak is present in the system.

Capacity of bag requires is based on body weight of patient as follow:

1. <15 lbs - 1 liter bag.
2. 15-40 lbs - 2 liter bag.
3. 40-120 lbs - 3 liter bag.

3. Pressure relief valve (pop-off valve)

Waste gases exit the anaesthetic circuit and enter the scavenging system at the pop-off valve. The valve prevents the buildup of excessive pressure or volume of gases within the circuit. It can be turned fully open, partly open or closed off entirely, allowing varying amounts of gas to exit the system. It is generally kept mostly open during anaesthesia, allowing gas to escape. The valve is then re-opened, again allowing the gases to vent. If valve was to remain closed, the excess pressure in the circuit would eventually reach the animal's lungs, causing alveoli to distend and possibly rupture.

4. Carbon dioxide absorbing canister

Any gases that do not exit the system through the pop-off valve are directed to the CO_2 absorber canister before being returned to the patient. The canister contains either soda lime or barium hydroxide lime. Calcium hydroxide in the absorbent removes carbon dioxide from the gases that percolate through the canister. Soda lime or barium hydroxide lime granules become exhausted after several hours of use and will no longer absorb CO_2. The use of depleted granules may result in excessive carbon dioxide delivery to the patient and hypercapnia.

Exhaustion of the granules can be indicated by several means which listed below.

- Color change (from white to blue or purple, depends on dye color). The color indicator reverts to its original color when not in use; therefore, exhausted granules should be changed immediately when noticed.

- Soft and crushable granules are converted to hard and non-crushable granules.

- Calcium hydroxide changes to calcium carbonate limestone.

- Generally granules are changed after every 8 hours of normal use.

5. Pressure manometer

Measures the pressure of the gases within the anaesthetic system (expressed in centimeters of water), which in turn reflects the pressure of gas in the animal's airway and lungs. Pressure over 15 cm of water indicate a build-up of air within the machine, either because the pop-off valve is closed or the oxygen flow rate is too high. When bagging an animal pressure should not exceed 15 to 20 cm H_2O. If a pressure manometer is not present, the anesthetist must rely on observation of the reservoir bag and patient to assess gas pressure. In this case, the reservoir bag should be compressed just enough to cause a slight rise in the patient's chest.

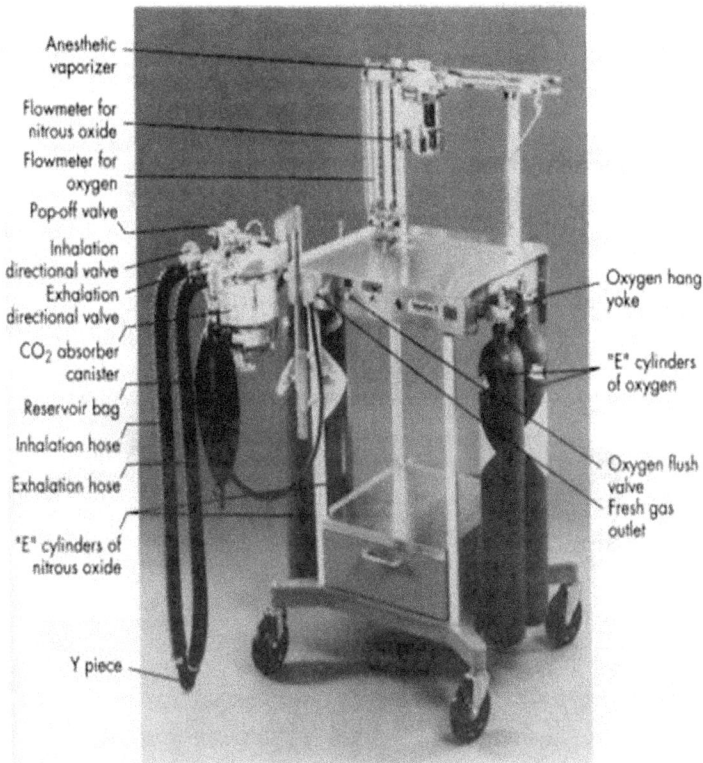

Figure 6.2: Anaesthetic machine (Boyle's apparatus)

Endotracheal intubation

Endotracheal intubation require for safe inhalation anaesthesia include establishment of patient airway with assurance of adequate ventilation and oxygenation.

Endotracheal intubation can be accomplished through

- Oral cavity
- Nasal passages
- An external pharyngeotomy or tracheotomy

Indication

1. Maintenance of a patient airway
2. Protection of airway from foreign material
3. Application of positive pressure ventilation
4. Application of tracheal or bronchial suction
5. For maintenance of anaesthesia
6. Administration of oxygen and inhalant anaesthetics

Advantage

1. Endotracheal intubation reduces anatomical dead space if the tube is correctly positioned and of the correct size.

2. For maintenance of anaesthesia endotracheal intubation create a seal with the trachea to prevent leakage of the anaesthetics gases into the environment.

Types of endotracheal tube

Two types of endotracheal tube are used in the veterinary practice:

1. Murphy type

Murphy tube has an opening which is known as Murphy eye or side hole, hole is located at the opposite the bevel and this hole allows gas flow even if the end hole is occluded. Murphy tube is cuff type tube and this tube use mostly in veterinary practice for which appropriate sizes are available.

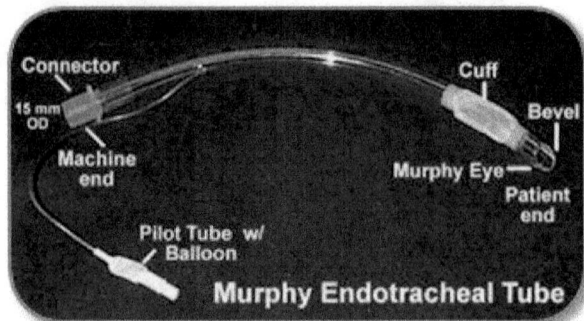

Figure 6.3: Murphy type

2. Cole type

Cole tubes are uncuffed and are characterized by a shoulder near the distal end. The diameter of patient end of the Cole tube is smaller than the reminder end of the Cole tube. Only the smaller portion of the tube should fit in to the tracheal and larynx, although fitting the sloping shoulder of the tube against the arytenoid cartilage create seal. To avoid pressure against the laryngeal cartilage and to prevent laryngeal dilation, the shoulder should not contact the larynx. The diameter of the tube should be such that the part of the tube creates seal, which prevent egress of gases and aspiration of foreign material.

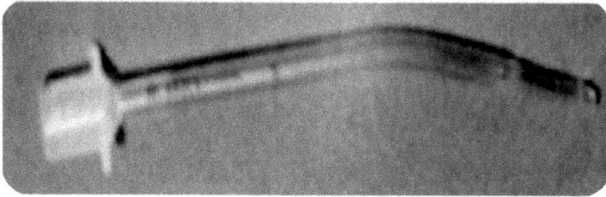

Figure 6.4: Cole type

Laryngoscope

A laryngoscope greatly facilitates the process of intubation in many animals and is a piece of equipment which is most desirable. A suitable laryngoscope usually holds a dry electric battery in the handle and has detachable blades of different sizes. The blades should be designed so as to enable the passage of a large bore endotracheal tube to be made as easily as possible.

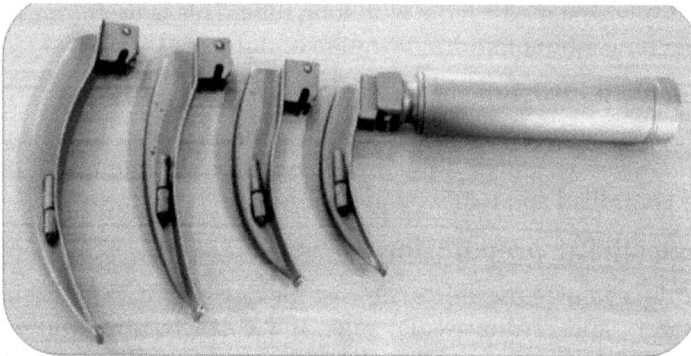

Figure 6.5: Laryngoscope with detachable blades

Other monitoring gadgets and equipments / instruments

1. Stethoscope

Use for auscultation of heart and lung sound.

2. Pulse oximeter

Use to monitor SPO_2 and pulse rate during the anaesthesia. Multiparameter monitor use to monitor ECG, respiration rate, pulse rate, blood pressure, SPO_2, temperature during the anaesthesia at a time.

3. Oxygen cylinder

Oxygen cylinders are coded with black colour. Two types of cylinders are used. Small cylinder fit into a yoke over pins which are indexed for different gases so as to make it impossible to attach an incorrect cylinder. Large cylinder utilizes 'bull-nose' fitting which screw into place and which require no sealing washer. A source of oxygen is required for inhalation anaesthetic apparatus.

4. Carbon dioxide cylinder

It is coated with gray colour. The CO_2 gas is compressed under a pressure which liquefies then at ordinary room temperature and kept in the cylinder. The amount of pressure can only be found by weighing. It is needed to be fitted with pressure regulators.

5. Nitrous oxide cylinder

This cylinder is coated with blue colour. The N_2O gas is compressed under a pressure which liquefies then at ordinary room temperature and kept in the cylinder. It is needed to be fitted with pressure regulators. It is a week anaesthetic drug used to supplement other drug.

6. Face mask

Administration of oxygen by means of a mask is effective during anaesthesia and for short periods during emergencies.

7. Scalp vein set

It is specifically designed needle with long tube. This is useful for fixing into superficial vein for continuous administration of fluid.

8. Continuous drip infusion set

This is specially designed set used for continuous drip infusion of anaesthetic solution for maintaining longer duration of anasthesia. A number of drops per minute can be controlled and total volume utilized can be measured.

Inhalant anaesthetic preparation

❖ Clinically evaluate the animal at least the day before anaesthesia. Record respiratory and cardiovascular rates and characteristics, pulse rate and characteristics, body weight, body temperature, capillary refill time and any abnormalities.

❖ Small animals should be fasted 12 hours and water withheld 6 hours, prior to induction of general anaesthesia.

❖ Plan, calculate and record the preanaesthetic and general anaesthetic regime, including dosage and volume of drugs to be administered.

❖ Assemble all supplies *i.e.*, needles, syringes, scalp vein, adhesive tape, saline flush, sponges, endotracheal tubes, roll gauze, lubricating jelly, ophthalmic ointment, etc.

- ❖ Prepare and label all drugs. Assemble and check all equipment (*i.e.* laryngoscope, anaesthesia machine, patient monitors, cautery, suction, etc.).

- ❖ Check to ensure that the control dial of the vaporizer is in the off position.

- ❖ Remove the filler cap by turning it counter-clockwise. If the vaporizer is pressurized, turn the cap slowly. Fill the vaporizer only with anaesthetic solution so that the fluid level reaches the upper line of the sight glass.

- ❖ Replace the cap by turning it clockwise. Check the colour and consistency of the carbon dioxide absorber. If half of the absorbent in the canister has changed colour, it should be replaced.

- ❖ Connect appropriate size breathing bag.

- ❖ Connect re-breathing circuit (for patients >5 lbs body weight) or Bain or Ayres T semi-open system (for patients <5 lbs body weight) to machine.

- ❖ Paediatric rebreathing hoses are recommended for patients <35 lbs body weight.

- ❖ The tank should be replaced when the pressure gauge registers less than 200 Psi. Reducing valve on machine lowers tank pressure to 50 Psi delivery pressure. A full tank will register 2000 Psi.

- ❖ Turn the oxygen flow meter on then off to check that the gas supply is operational.

- ❖ Open and close the "pop-off" pressure relief valve to make sure it is working freely. Depress and release the oxygen flush valve. Pressure check the circuit by closing the "pop-off" pressure relief valve and covering the patient opening of the Y-piece on the end of the circuit hose.

- ❖ Activate the oxygen flush until the system pressure level reads 20 cm H_2O. Hold this position for a few seconds.

- ❖ If there are no leaks, the pressure will hold steady. If the pressure drops, open the oxygen flow meter until the pressure stabilizes at 20 cm H_2O. If more than 300 ml/min of oxygen is required to stabilize the system pressure at 20 cm H_2O, the leak is of a great enough magnitude to justify servicing. Identify leaks using water or soapy solutions and conduct repairs.

Endotracheal intubation in dogs

Preparation

- ❖ Select several endotracheal tubes of varying sizes and check them for leaks, holes or loose connectors.

- ❖ Determine appropriate length of the tube requires. By measuring the distance from the incisors to the thoracic inlet. Properly placed, the end of the tube should be half way between the larynx and the thoracic inlet.

❖ When the animal reaches an appropriate plane of anaesthesia, open the mouth to allow intubation.

❖ The animal should not be showing any signs of resistance. The animal is restrained in sternal recumbency with the head and neck extended in a straight line. The restrainer should hold the upper jaw stationary with the lips pulled dorsally and pull the lower jaw down by pulling the tongue forward and down.

❖ The restrainer should not push on the animal's ventral neck as this may obscure the laryngeal anatomy. All patients should be intubated with the largest endotracheal tube that fits comfortably in the trachea. Resistance to respiration is determined primarily by the diameter of the endotracheal tube. Larger tube shows less resistance.

Intubation

A laryngoscope can be used to assist intubation by illuminating the pharyngeal area and moving the epiglottis aside to allow visualization of the glottis. The laryngoscope blade is first used to disengage the soft palate from the epiglottis, and then gently placed at the back of the tongue to pull the epiglottis forward. Successful passage of the tube is enhanced by proper depth of anaesthesia, correct positioning, use of a laryngoscope (especially as a light source), a proper size endotracheal tube and a judicious amount of sterile lubricant. Endotracheal tube is introducing by open the mouth and progress it through trachea after pull down the epiglottis cartilage. Following intubation, correct placement can be confirmed by mild cough, feeling air coming out of the endotracheal tube in synchrony of movement of the chest. The tube should not be forced through the vocal cords, but gently rotated, if resistance is encountered. Non-traumatic intubation is very important. Endotracheal tube sizes are proportional to the body weight, typically using 8-12 mm for average 12-24 kg dogs. With smaller tubes, a polypropylene urinary catheter can be used as a stylet to provide more rigidity and allow easier intubation. If a stylet is used, the tip of the stylet should not protrude past the tip of the tube to avoid damage to the trachea. Ensure that the tube enters the trachea and not the esophagus. If cannot visualize the tube entering the trachea, do not assume it is in place. Double check or re-intubate.

Other ways to verify proper placement

1. Cough reflex
2. Feel air passing through tube when animal breathes
3. Visualize reservoir bag and unidirectional valves moving during respiration
4. Palpate a single firm tube in throat
5. Vocalization is impossible with tube correctly placed

Secure the tube in place with a piece of gauze tied around the tube and behind the animal's head or on top of the muzzle.

Cuff inflation

Before inflating the cuff of the endotracheal tube, check for leakage of anaesthetic gas around the cuff by gently squeezing the reservoir bag and listening for air around the tube. If the tube is of an appropriate size, one does not hear a leak and are able to adequately ventilate the patient. If the cuff needs to be inflated, ventilate the patient while adding air slowly to the cuff. The cuff should be inflated just until no longer hear a loud hiss of air around the tube. Over-inflation of the cuff can result in necrosis and sloughing of the tracheal lining. The subjective feel of the inflation balloon is not an acceptable method of evaluating the cuff.

Chapter 7

Intravenous General Anaesthesia

Preanaesthetic preparation

The preanaesthetic examination or evaluation will influence greatly on the dose and choice of the premedicants, induction agents and maintenance agents as well as selection of anaesthetic techniques. Thorough patient evaluation and preparation will improve patient safety and ensure successful anaesthetic outcome.

Preparation of the patient

Food and water withholding time

- Varies between species
- Dogs and cats: usually 12 hours and minimum of 6 hours.
- Large ruminants (cattle and buffaloes): Roughage for 24 hours.
- Small ruminants (sheep and goats) and calves: Feed and roughages for 12-24 hours.
- Horses: Roughage and concentrates for 24 hours.
- Neonatal patient must not be starved because of their high metabolic demands, and to prevent susceptible hypoglycemia.
- Free access to water right up to premedication in small animal.
- In ruminant 6 hour water withholding time for prevention of regurgitation.

Fluid and electrolytes

- Correct dehydrated patient using isotonic saline, Ringer lactate or supplement deficient electrolytes or correct excessive electrolytes.
- Stabilization of the patient in the fluid balance and electrolyte imbalance will substantially reduce deranged physiology during anaesthesia.
- Volume depletion during the anaesthesia will be less if adequate time is spent prior to the induction increasing the chance of survival.

- Unless life threatening and the animal can wait until fluid imbalance can be corrected, it is not recommended to subject the animal for general anaesthesia.

History

- Nature and duration of illness: Acute or chronic, the severity of the illness.
- Any previous anaesthetic episodes.
- Past and current medications.
- Concurrent of secondary disease: Diarrhea, vomiting (fluid imbalance)

Physical examination

- *Body condition:* obesity, cachexia, dehydration.
- Temperature, heart rate and respiratory rate.
- Auscultate the heart and lung and note any unusual characteristics and if necessary postpone the anaesthesia until fully clear the questionable condition.
- *Cardiopulmonary system:* heart rate and rhythm, auscultate the characteristics, capillary refill time, color of mucous membrane, exercise intolerance, coughing, dyspnea.
- *CNS and special senses:* Temperament, seizure, coma, stupor, ataxia, vision and hearing impairment.
- *Gastrointestinal:* Auscultate the gut sound, parasites, palpation.
- *Hepatic:* Icterus, abnormal bleeding.
- *Renal:* Palpate kidneys and bladder, polyuria / polydipsia, oliguria.
- *Integument:* Tumors and flea infestation.
- *Musculoskeletal:* Fractures, deformity and lameness

Laboratory investigation

Minimum data base

1. Packed cell volume (PCV).
2. Total plasma protein (TPP).
3. Blood urea nitrogen (BUN).
4. Glucose.

These four tests should be performed on all patients.

Other diagnostics, as indicated by physical examination and history

1. Radiography
2. Echocardiography
3. Ultrasonography

Classification of the Physical Status (adopted by the American Society of Anesthesiologists, ASA)

a) Normal healthy patient (neutering, ovariohysterectomy)

b) Mild to moderate systemic disease (cruciate rupture repair, laryngeal hemiplegia repair)

c) Severe systemic disease. Severe dehydration (portosystemic shunt disease, compensated renal insufficiency)

d) Severe systemic disease that is a constant threat to life (Gastric dilatation and volvulus, equine colic, dystocia)

e) Moribund, not expected to live 24 hours irrespective of intervention (ruptured arteries)

f) Emergency surgery

Total Intra-Venous Anaesthesia (TIVA)

Most commonly employed TIVA is based on balanced anaesthetic combination. It can be used to induce anaesthesia with a single bolus dose, and then to maintain anaesthesia using constant rate infusion. Recovery is very smooth and complete even following prolonged use. Different combinations are associated with minimal cardiopulmonary depression. However, there are two main limitations to continued administration of intravenous anaesthetics; the arterial oxygenation and prolonged recovery. Arterial oxygenation is always at risk with TIVA, particularly with combination of propofol and opioids. Anaesthetic depth control is more difficult with TIVA so abrupt awakening during anaesthesia is more likely if one is not familiar with the technique.

Anaesthetic Combinations used in Small and Large Animals

1. Thiopental Sodium

It is a commonly used general anaesthetic, which produces anaesthesia of very short duration. It is available in yellow colour powder form (0.5 and 1.0 g vials) and should be freshly prepared (2.5 to 10 per cent) in distilled water or physiological saline, but never in dextrose/dextrose saline. It is used preferably after premedication to avoid complications during anaesthesia and recovery. It induces anaesthesia rapidly on intravenous administration. A 25-50 per cent of calculated dose is given according to condition of patient in 5-10 seconds followed by a pause of 30-45 seconds so as to recover from barbiturate apnoea followed by intermittent dosing to abolish pedal reflex.

Dose

Dog and Cat: 20-25 mg/kg IV for 10 to 20 minutes of surgical anaesthesia without premedication, when induction is proceed by preanaesthetic sedation; a dose range of 6 to 10 mg/kg is used.

Large animals: 1g/90 kg (5-10 per cent).

2. Ketamine and Xylazine anaesthesia in Equine

Dose: Xylazine 1.1 mg/kg IV produce head tilting of animal within five-ten minutes followed by injection of Ketamine HCl 2.2 mg/kg IV will produce balance anaesthesia.

3. Ketamine – diazepam combination used in canines

Dose: Ketamine HCl 5 mg/kg and Diazepam 0.5 mg/kg combination is taken to induce as well as maintenance of anaesthsia by intravenous route.

4. Propofol

It is used in dogs and horses. It will produce smooth induction of anaesthesia. It can be used in combination of Acepromazine.

Dose: Horse- 2 mg/kg IV

Dog- 4-6 mg/kg IV

Chapter 8

Anaesthetic Emergencies

Surgeon should have proper knowledge about stages of general anaesthesia for better management of general anaesthesia and anaesthetic emergencies.

Stages of general anaesthesia

Stage I   :   Induction stage / stage of voluntary excitement.

Stage II   :   Stage of involuntary excitement.

Stage III   :   Stage of surgical anaesthesia

             i. First plane (Light anaesthesia)

             ii. Second plane (Medium anaesthesia)

             iii. Third plane (Deep anaesthesia)

Stage IV   :   Over dosage or stage of medullary paralysis.

Monitoring of the Patient

Anaesthetic monitoring is an important to maintain a proper plane of anesthesia and to prevent excessive insult to the cardiovascular, respiratory and central nervous systems.

Anaesthetic depth can be measured by following observations

- Physical movement or jaw chewing in response to stimulation, eye position and degree of muscle tone, and presence or absence of palpebral reflexes etc.

- Variables used to monitor the cardiovascular system include heart rate, blood pressure, mucous membrane colour and capillary refill time.

- Direct blood pressure measurement can provide continuous hemodynamic status of the animal and can be easily accomplished through catheterizing the auricular artery.

- The ECG is useful to monitor cardiac dysrhythmias.

- The respiratory system is evaluated by monitoring respiratory rate and volume.
- It can be estimated by observing the emptying of the rebreathing bag of the anaesthetic machine during respiratory cycles.
- Pulse oximetry and/or arterial blood gas analysis provide information of the ventilatory efficiency
- Ocular reflexes are used to monitor the central nervous system. The palpebral reflex is lost at light planes of anaesthesia in ruminants, so it is of little value during anaesthesia of these species.
- Body temperature is also an important parameter to monitor during anesthesia. Body temperature must be maintained so as not to prolong the recovery, and lessen oxygen requirement by muscle tissues.

Anaesthetic Emergencies and its Management

1. Respiratory insufficiency and arrest

- Supply oxygen through ventilator
- Use respiratory analeptic – Doxapram 2 mg/kg IV

2. Cardiovascular Insufficiency and Arrest

- Supply oxygen through ventilator
- Closed thoracic cardiac massage
- Inj. Sodium bicarbonate 25 mEq/10 kg IV
- Inj. Epinephrine (1 : 10000) 0.5 – 2 ml Intracardiac
- Calcium gluconate 5–10 ml of 10 per cent solution IV
- Calcium chloride 1–3 ml of 10 per cent solution IV
- Inj. Lidocaine 1 mg/kg – To correct bradycardia

3. Regurgitation and Vomition

- Proper intubation followed by inflation of cuff
- Sternal recumbency with head down is preferred in ruminants
- Oxygen supply should be continued

4. Anaesthetic Overdose

- Fluid therapy
- Proper antidote
- Hyper ventilation and controlled supply of inhalant anaesthesia

5. Temperature Regulation

- Maintain warm and comfort environment of operation theatre
- IV fluid being administered should be warmed to body temperature

Chapter 9

Local and Regional Anaesthesia

Local analgesia (anaesthesia): It is loss of sensation in a limited body area.

Primarily used in cattle, buffalo, sheep, goats and equines depending upon the co-operative nature of the patient.

Advantages

- Minimal equipment needed.
- Minimal systemic effects.

Disadvantages

- Require co-operative patient with or without significant restraint
- May be require sedation

Types of local anaesthetic techniques

1. Topical or surface anaesthesia

This technique is primarily used to desensitize superficial layer of skin/mucous membrane *i.e.* eye, glans penis, vulvar lips etc.

a. Using volatile agents

These agents evaporate instantly thereby decreasing the surface temperature and so causing desensitization of area. It should not be used frequently otherwise it will cause tissue necrosis *e.g.* Ethyl chloride spray, ether spray.

b. Using local anaesthetics

Lignocaine HCl (2 per cent) is used for the relief of pain in the abrasion or eczematous area. Sock a piece of cotton or gauge in local anaesthetic solution and then put on the affected area for five minutes. The analgesia is produced for 30-45 minutes.

2. Infiltration anaesthesia

It affects nerve endings at the actual site of operation. Most of the minor surgical operation can be performed under infiltration anaesthesia and the technique is also useful in conjunction with light basal narcosis for major operations in animals which are at poor surgical risks. Amount of local anaesthesia depends upon body area of animal as well as part to be operated.

Indication

It is used to desensitize the nerve endings of operative field.

Types of extra vascular infiltration anaesthesia

i. Linear infiltration

It means that deposition of local anaesthetic along the line of incision. A needle about 10 cm long is introduced almost parallel to the skin surface and pushed through subcutaneous tissue along the proposed line. Before injecting any local analgesic solution, aspiration is attempted to ascertain that the needle point has not entered a blood vessel.

ii. Field block

Local anaesthetics agent is infiltrated in such a way that they make wall of analgesia enclosing the site of incision.

a) Diamond Block

The local anaesthetic are infiltrated linearly around the periphery of the site in a diamond shaped manner. This is used in the case of tumour excision and lymph node biopsy.

b) Inverted 'L' block

A local anaesthetic is injected into the tissues bordering the dorso-caudal aspect of the last rib and ventro-lateral aspect of the lumbar transverse process. This is used for a rumenotomy. About 10-15 min is required for the onset of the analgesic effect.

c) 'T' block

It is similar to the inverted 'L' block, wherein the local anaesthetic is infiltrated in the manner of a "T" shape.

iii. Ring block

Analgesia of the foot and the teat can be produced by ring block. It is a special type of block, in which local anaesthetic is deposited in a transverse plane through the whole extremities. For analgesia of the foot, local anaesthetics solution is deposited in the tissue around the limb at the middle third of the metatarsus or the metacarpus. Infiltration of the local anaesthetics in the skin and muscle of the teat base, around its entire circumference provides adequate analgesia to the teat.

Advantage

Require no greater skill or the knowledge of the anatomy of the part to be operated.

Disadvantage

- Large volume of local anaesthetic is required.
- Epinephrine in local anaesthetic may lead to delayed healing as well as restrict blood supply.

3. Intravenous Regional Anaesthsia (IVRA)

Indication

To produce regional anaesthesia of lower limb, especially for surgery of digits.

Procedure

Secure the animal in lateral recumbency with the limb to be anaesthestised in lower most position. Then tourniquet applies above the site of insertion leads to engorgement of vein. Ten to twenty ml of local anaesthetic is injected via the needle in the vein in bovines and five ml in small ruminant.

Advantage

Analgesia of the limb up to the lower limit of the tourniquet comes on rapidly in about 10 minutes and once tourniquet released it wears off with almost equal rapidity.

Disadvantage

Longer procedure leads to tissue hypoxia and severe lameness.

4. Peripheral nerve block

It involves injection of local anaesthetic solution around a sensory nerve trunk.

A. Peterson's orbital nerve block

Indications

Surgical management of eye ball, eye lid and horns.

Site

At the foramen orbitorotundum from where third (oculomotor), fourth (trochlear), sixth (abducens) and ophthalmic and maxillary parts of fifth (trigeminal) cranial nerves emerge.

Procedure

A 12 cm long 18 G needle is then inserted from the same space and pushed till it strikes the coronoid process of the mandible. Then it is redirected towards the pterygopalatine fossa rostal to the foramen orbitorotundum, at the depth of 8 to 10 cm. At this site 15- 20 ml of 2 per cent lignocaine is injected.

B. Auriculopalpebral nerve block

Indications

1. To relieve the spasm of eye lid following an eye injury.

2. Management of surgical condition of eye lid and eye ball in conjunction with the retrobulbar nerve block.

3. For examination of eye.

Site

Three cm below the highest point of the dorsal border of the zygomatic arch.

Procedure

Three cm long 16 G needle is first inserted through skin at the depression for skin weal just caudal to the point where the supra orbital process meets the zygomatic arch. A 12 cm long 18 G needle is then inserted from the same space and pushed obliquely and dorsally to contact the bone and pushed along the bone until the point almost reaches the border of zygomatic arch below 3 cm level and inject 5 to 7 ml of Lignocaine HCl (2 per cent) at the site.

C. Mental nerve block

Indications

Surgery of lower lip and lower jaw including gums and mandible.

Site

At lateral aspect of ramus just behind the fourth incisor.

Procedure

Three - four cm long 20 G needle, slightly bent is inserted in the foramen and 15-20 ml of 2 per cent lignocaine is injected. Same procedure is repeated on other side of the mandible.

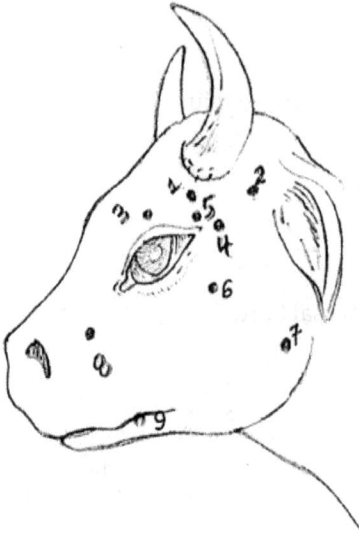

1. Auriculopalpebral nerve block
2. Cornual nerve block
3. Supra orbital nerve block
4. Peterson's orbital nerve block
5. Retrobulbar nerve block
6. Maxillary nerve block
7. Mandibular nerve block
8. Infraorbital nerve block
9. Mental nerve block

Figure 9.1: Head region nerve block in cattle

D. Mandibulo–alveolar nerve block

Indication

Surgery of molar teeth, incisors and lower lip.

Site

At mandibular foramen at medial aspect of ramus of mandible.

Procedure

A 15 cm long 18 G needle is inserted at the angle of jaw along the medial surface of ramus of mandible, at a point where an imaginary line along the masticatory surface of the lower molar teeth is crossed by another vertical line from the lateral canthus of the eye. About 20 ml of 2 per cent of lignocaine is injected at the site to produce analgesia.

E. Caudal epidural analgesia

Indications

i. Posterior block/Low epidural block

1. Surgical operations on the tail.
2. Suturing of the tears of the perineum and vulva.
3. Surgical manipulations of the anus.
4. Examination of the vagina.
5. To control straining.

6. Manipulation and correction of malpresentation of foetus during delivery.

7. Reduction of vaginal and uterine prolapse.

8. Treatment of parturient injuries.

9. Simple embryotomy operations.

10. Ovariectomy.

ii. Anterior block/High epidural block

1. Examination and operations of the penis.

2. Cutting operations on the prepuce and inguinal regions.

3. Castration.

4. Operative interferences on the udder.

5. Operations on the hind limb.

6. Extensive embryotomy.

7. Amputation of uterus.

8. Caesarean section.

Restraint

Standing position with the animal secured in a travis

Site

At the space between the arches of first and second coccygeal vertebrae.

Procedure

The tail is gripped about 6″ from its base and raised 'pump handle' fashion. The tip of the thumb is then passed backwards from the spine of the sacrum. The next prominence to be felt is the spine of the first coccygeal vertebra. The site is the depression immediately behind it. At this site, first, an insensitive skin weal is made. The point of needle is then applied at the centre of this depression. The needle is thrust downwards and forwards at an angle of 15 degree to the vertical until its point impinges on the floor of the canal. It is slightly withdrawn and 5 to 10 ml of 2 per cent solution of local anaesthetic is injected slowly. If the needle is correctly in the epidural space there will be no resistance on the plunger and the solution goes easily in the canal. This results into posterior block desensitising tail, croup as far as mid-sacral region, anus, vulva, perineum and posterior aspect of the thighs.

The onset of analgesia within 5 to 10 minutes and the analgesia remains for about 45 to 60 minutes.

Dose

Anterior block is achieved through the same site. However, the dose rate differs. It varies between 30 to 150 ml depending upon the size of the animal and the type of the operation to be performed. For difficult embryotomy, examination of penis, open method of castration, etc. 40 to 80 ml, and for caesarean section, amputation of udder, operations on the hind limbs, amputation of uterus, etc. 60 to 120 ml lignocain HCl (2 per cent) solution can be used.

F. Paravertebral analgesia

The block results into a uniform anaesthesia of the respective para-lumbar fossa. The surgical interferences involving the opening of the flank can be undertaken with this block; viz., rumenotomy and correction of left displacement of abomasum on the left side as well as all the surgical interferences of the intestine on the right side.

Restraint

Standing position with the animal secured in a travis.

Site

The procedure involves blocking the 13th thoracic, 1st, 2nd and 3th lumbar nerves. For blocking the 13th thoracic spinal nerve, the injection is made just behind the head of last rib. To determine the sites for lumbar nerves, a transverse line is drawn immediately behind the spinous process of the particular vertebra and the needle is inserted at a point on this line 5 cm from the mid-line. The nerves lie at a depth of about 5 cm.

Procedure

An insensitive skin weal is first produced at the predetermined sites, using a short (3 cm) 20 gauge needle by injecting about 3 ml of 2 per cent local anaesthetic solution. After an appropriate pause, for blocking the 13th thoracic spinal nerve, an 18 gauge, 8 cm long needle is inserted directly downwards, through the selected site, till the needle strikes the anterior edge of the transverse process of the 1st lumbar vertebra. It is then redirected a little forward and deeper just in front of the process. At this point 5 to 10 ml of lignocain (2 per cent) solution are injected. During withdrawal of the needle a further 5 ml are infiltrated along the track. During the final withdrawal of the needle, the skin is pressed downwards to prevent separation of the connective tissue and aspiration of the air through the needle.

For blocking 1st, 2nd and 3rd lumbar spinal nerves a similar procedure is adopted through respective sites. However, the needle point strikes the anterior edge of the transverse process of the next lumbar vertebra. Then it is directed little forward and deeper so as to penetrate the inter-transverse ligament. At this point the anaesthetic solution is deposited as describe earlier. The onset of analgesia of the flank is within 5 to 10 minutes and the effect remains for about 60 minutes.

G. Field block - Rumenotomy

Indication

Laparotomy through left paralumber fossa.

Restraint

Standing animal secured in a travis.

Site

Left paralumber fossa.

Procedure

A 18 gauge, 15 cm long needle is inserted in the skin about 5 cm below the transverse process of the 3rd lumbar vertebra. It is then directed anteriorly so that the needle lies under the skin. The anaesthetic solution (2 per cent) is then deposited while slowly withdrawing the needle. The rate is approximately 1 ml of the solution for every cm of withdrawal the needle is then directed into the abdominal musculature up to the peritoneum. The procedure of injection is again repeated. Now the needle is directed posteriorly and above procedure of injection, both under the skin and into the musculature are again repeated. Now the needle is directed downward so as to lie, first under the skin and the anaesthetic solution is deposited as described above, similarly the anaesthetic solution is deposited into the musculature up to the peritoneum. The procedure results into a "T" shaped block completely desensitizing the paralumber fossa. The onset is within 5 to 10 minutes and the effect remains for about 60 minutes.

H. Lumbar epidural analgesia

The procedure results into belt of analgesia around the animal's trunk without interfering control of hind limbs. Hence, under this block laparotomy through both the flanks and also through the ventral abdominal region can be performed.

Restraint

Standing position with the animal secured in the travis.

Site

Just to the right of the lumbar spinous processes on a line 1.5 cm behind the anterior edge of the second lumbar transverse process.

Procedure

An initial skin weal is made with a fine needle at the site. A 18 gauge 12 cm long needle is then introduced and directed downward and inward at an angle of 10-30 degree with the vertical, for a distance of about 7.5 cm. At this point the needle has entered the spinal canal. If the needle is correctly in the epidural space, air enters the canal making hissing sound. Now about 7 to 10 ml of 2 per cent anaesthetic solution is injected. The needle is withdrawn by pressing the skin. The onset of analgesia is within about 10 minutes and the effect remains for about 3 hours.

I. Infra orbital nerve block

Indications

For surgical interference of upper lip, cheek, nostrils and lower parts of the face when the nerve is blocked outside the canal. If the nerve is blocked in the canal then surgical intervention involving 1st and 2nd premolar, incisor teeth of that side inclusive of their alveoli and contiguous gums can be under taken.

Restraint

Standing position or lateral recumbency.

Site

Just at the level of the 1st premolar *i.e.* below and medial to the facial tuberosity. At this site the lip of the foramen can be palpated.

Procedure

The injection can be made at two places. First injection is at the foramen as the nerve emerges out of the infra-orbital canal and the second into the infra-orbital canal. The lip of the foramen is palpated and a skin weal is made at the site. The weal is necessary if the injection is to be made into the canal. An 18 gauge 2" long needle is inserted and about 4 to 5 ml of 2 per cent anaesthetic solution is injected just in front *i.e.* below the bony lip of the canal. If the injection is to be made into the canal then the needle is held parallel to the skin and introduced about 2 to 2.5 cm deep into the canal. Here another 4 to 5 ml of anaesthetic solution is deposited. The analgesia takes effect within 5 to 10 minutes and effect remains for about 45 to 60 minutes.

J. Cornual nerve block

Indication

Surgical interferences of the horn.

Restraint

Standing position, or lateral recumbency depending on the type of surgical interference.

Site

At the upper third of the temporal ridge and about 2.5 cm below the base of the horn; the needle is inserted so that its point lies 0.7 to 1 cm deep, immediately behind the ridge.

Procedure

A skin weal is made at the site. After sufficient pause an 18 gauge 5 cm long needle is inserted at the determined site and 1 ml of anaesthetic solution is injected. The needle should not be inserted too deeply, otherwise injection will be made beneath the aponeurosis of the temporal muscle and the method will fail, In large horned animals it is advisable that a second injection is made about 1 cm behind the first to block the posterior division of the nerve. Loss of sensation develops within 10 to 15 minutes and lasts about one hour.

K. Retrobulbar analgesia

Indication

Enucleation of the eyeball.

Restraint

Lateral recumbency.

Site

About 2 to 2.5 cm lateral to the lateral canthus of the eye.

Procedure

A skin weal is prepared 2 to 2.5 cm lateral to the lateral canthus of the eye. A 10 cm long 18 G needle is introduced through the weal and directed inward and slightly forward through the temporal fossa till the needle edge touch opposite wall of the orbital cavity. It is then slightly withdrawn and 30 ml of 2 per cent local anaesthetic solution is deposited. On completion of the injection the eyeball slightly protrude out.

L. Spermatic nerve block

Castration.

Restraint

Lateral recumbency casting by castration method.

Site

In to the spermatic cord about 2.5 cm above the base of the scrotum.

Procedure

The lower testicle is held taut and the spermatic cord is palpated. A short 18-gauge needle is introduced in the structures of the spermatic cord and 10 ml of 2 per cent local anaesthetic solution is deposited. The procedure is repeated on the other testicle. In case of open method of castration in addition to the spermatic block few milliliters of 2 per cent anaesthetic solution is injected also into the testicular mass.

Chapter 10

Chemical Restraint of Laboratory and Wild Animals

General Consideration for Lab Animals

Animals are prepared for anaesthesia by overnight fasting. Atropine is most commonly used as an anti-cholinergic agent. Local or general anaesthesia may be used, depending on the type of surgical procedure. Local anaesthetics are used to block the nerve supply to a limited area only for minor operations. Anaesthetic agents generally affect cardiovascular, respiratory and thermoregulatory mechanism in addition to central nervous system. It should be carried out under expert supervision for regional infiltration of surgical site, nerve blocks, epidural and spinal anaesthesia.

A number of general anaesthetic agents are used in the form of inhalants, intravenous or intra-muscular injections. Species characteristics and variation must be kept in mind while using an anaesthetic. Side-effects such as excessive salivation, convulsions, excitement and disorientation should be suitably prevented and controlled.

Table: 10.1 Commonly used anaesthetic drugs for laboratory animals

Drugs (mg/kg)	Mouse	Rat	Hamster	Guinea	Rabbit	Cat	Dog	Monkey
Keteamine HCI (IM)	22–24	22–24	-	22–24	22–24	30	30	15–40
Pentobarbitone Sodium (IV)	35	25	35	30	30	25	25–30	35
Thiopentone Sodium (IV)	25	20	20	20	20	25	25	25

Chemical immobilization of wild animals

Wild animals are chemically restrained for the following reasons.

1. Animal translocation and transportation.
2. To study the ecology and population estimate.
3. For veterinary studies.
4. To relieve wild animals in distress to the public.

Various devices used for injecting the drug from a distance are dart guns, projectile syringes (short range, long range and extra long range), blowgun rifle, blowpipe and stick syringe.

Table: 10.2 Commonly Employed Anaesthetics in Different Wild Animal

Animal	Drug and dose
Primates:	Ketamine - 5-20 mg/kg intramuscular
	Xylazine 2mg/kg -intramuscular
Chimpanzee:	Ketamine - 10-15 mg/kg intramuscular
	Xylazine 2mg/kg -intramuscular
Kangaroo:	Xylazine 8 mg/kg
	Ketamine 3 mg/kg combination, intramuscular
Antelope:	Xylazine 0.23 mg/kg
	Ketamine 11.54 mg/kg combination, intramuscular
Deer:	Xylazine – 2.0 to 8.0 mg/kg
	Ketamine - 10-20 mg/kg intramuscular
Camels:	Xylazine - 0.27 to 0.51 mg/kg
Bears:	Xylazine 2-4 mg/kg
	Eetamine 4.5-9 mg/kg, combination, intramuscular
Bioson:	Chloral hydrate 250 mg/kg
Elephants:	Asian elephants 100-175 mg - Xylazine (Total dose)
	Etorphine- Acepromazine combination (2.4 mg/ml
	Etorphine, 10 mg/ml of Acepromazine per ml. Dose 1 ml/4 feet of shoulder height
Reptiles:	Ketamine 20 mg/kg intramuscular, Xylazine 1 mg/kg -intramuscular
Snakes:	Ketamine - 50-130 mg/kg intramuscular
	Tiletamine - 10-20-2mg/kg intramuscular

Chapter 11

X-Ray Equipment and Safety Measures in Radiography

X-ray machine

1. Fixed X-ray machine

These are suitable for almost all types of radiographic examination of large animals. A ceiling mounted telescoping tube support facilitates movement of the tube across the room and almost to the level of ground, apart from both horizontal and vertical X-ray beams. The output varies from 120-300 kV and 300-1000 mA. Exposure time is less, because of high kV and mA output. More scatter radiation occurs due to higher kV output and three phase electricity is required for installation.

2. Mobile X-ray machine

Most machines are movable on smooth surface within the radiology section. They are mounted on wheels and cumbersome to use for restless animals. Usually these machines have rotating anode. The output varies from 90-125 kV and 40-300 mA.

3. Portable X-ray machine

These machines are equipped with small sized low weight transformer located within the tube head. A small control panel is attached to the tube stand. The maximum output varies from 70-110 kV and 15-35 mA. These machines have stationary anode with both single and double focal spot and suitable for X-ray of limbs below stifle and elbow of large animals and can be used for taking X-rays of abdomen and skeletal systems of small animals. These machines are commonly used in veterinary practice because of their convenient transportation.

X-ray accessories in radiography

1. Lead aprons and gloves

The persons involved in radiography work must wear protective gloves and aprons. The protective gloves should have at least 0.5 mm lead equivalent whereas lead aprons should have minimum of 0.25 mm lead equivalent but 0.5 mm is preferred.

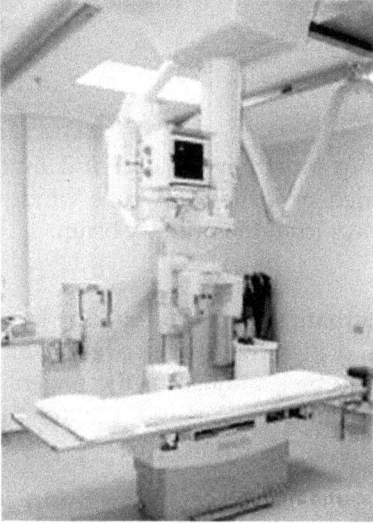

1. Fix x- ray machine

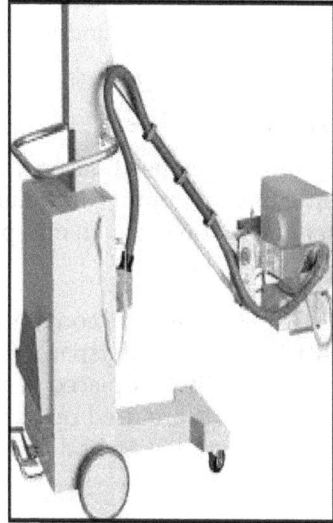

2. Mobile x-ray

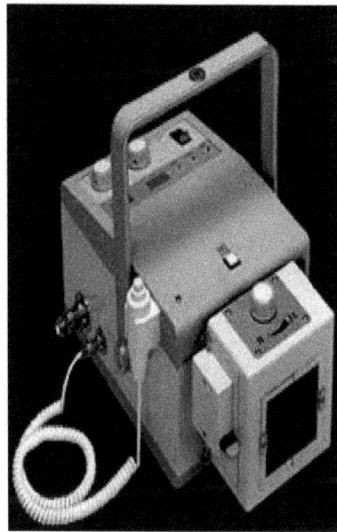

3. Portable x-ray

Figure 11.1: Different X- ray machines

2. Collimators

Collimation refers to the regulation of X-ray beam by beam restricting devices to restrict it to the site of the part of the patient under examination. It reduces scatter radiation.

Types of collimators

- Aperture diaphragm
- Cones and cylinders
- Variable aperture collimator.

3. Aluminum filter

X-ray machines that operate above 70 kVp must have a total of 2.5 mm of aluminium filtration. Aluminium filter is added over the X-ray tube window to filter out all useless, soft, non-penetrating X-rays from the primary beam.

4. Grid

Grid is a flat plate containing series of alternating strips of radiodense (Lead) and radiolucent (Interspacer) material encased in a protective covering of thin aluminium. Grid is placed between the part to be examined of the patient and cassette. Grids are used on parts more than 10 cm thick to reduce the fog caused by scattered radiation and to improve the radiographic detail.

Types of grids

- Parallel grid.
- Crossed grid.
- Focused grid.
- Moving grid.

5. Potter bucky diaphragm

A potter-bucky diaphragm is a grid that moves during a radiographic exposure to eliminate the grid lines on X-ray film produced by a stationary grid. It is not effective for less than 1/60 second exposures.

6. Cassettes

Cassettes are light proof boxes designed to hold the film and intensifying screen with good contact.

7. Intensifying screen

The intensifying screen consists of a uniform homogenous coating of minute tungstate crystals mounted on a plastic base, which intensifies the effect of X-rays.

8. X-ray films

X-ray films are available in various sizes. The standard sizes such as 17" x 14", 15" x 12", 12" x 10" and 10" x 8" are used routinely in veterinary practice. The film is made of transparent polyester base coated with an emulsion of silver halide crystals and gelatin.

Two types of X-ray films are used in diagnostic radiology.

i. Screen type.   ii. Non screen type.

9. X-ray film hanger

These are used for holding the exposed X-ray film during dark room processing and drying.

Three types of hangers are available.

i.   Channel type.
ii. Tension type.
iii. Clip type.

10. Cassette holder and block

Cassette holders have been designed with long handles to keep the individual holding the cassette well outside the primary beam. They are used in radiography of extremities of large animals. Blocks are usually necessary for large animal radiography to elevate an animal's foot to the centre of the X-ray beam. These blocks can be specially built or made from large pieces of wood.

11. Lead/film markers

These are used for identification of the view and case number. These lead letters or numbers can be attached to the name plate. This identification requires an assortment of small, inexpensive, lead numbers. Additional radiographic markers of equal importance are 'right', 'left' and 'lateral' aspect markers. Such markers are quite important in extremity radiographs, particularly for large animals.

12. Illuminator or viewer

These are used for viewing the developed X-ray film for interpretation.

These may be:

i. Fixed type.
ii. Revolving type.

13) X-ray film drier

It is used for drying the film after processing.

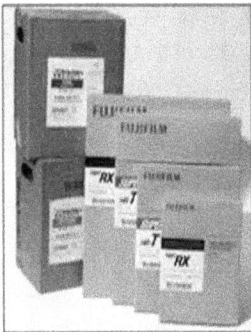 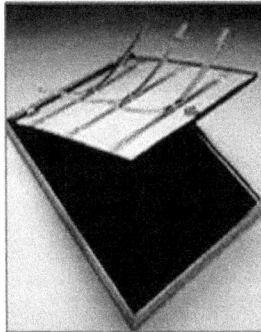 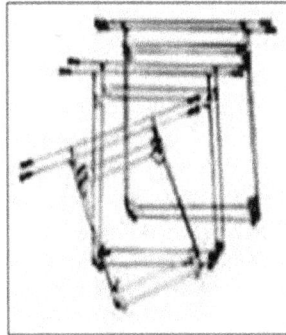

1. Film Storage box   2. Grid   3. Film Hanger

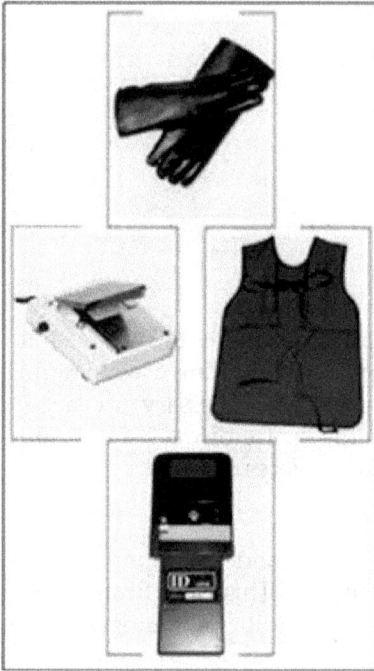

4. Gloves, Apron, Dryer

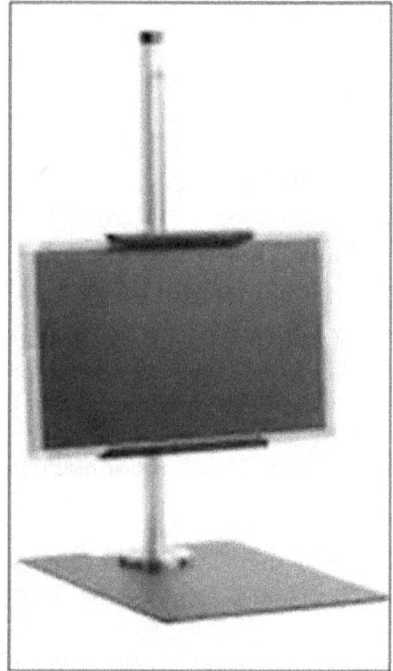

5. Cassette and Holder

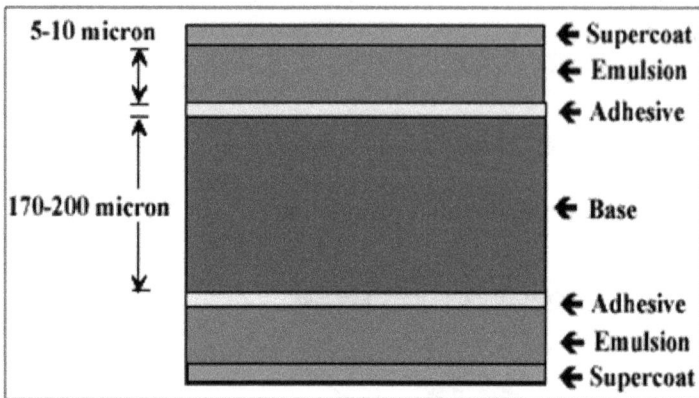

6. Cross-section through a double emulsion film

Figure 11.2: X- ray accessories.

Chapter 12

Dark Room Technique

Dark room has sufficient space to accommodate a dry bench and a wet section of same dimension and a sink. Room should be near to the X-ray examination area. Walls should be solid concrete and have lead boxes of unexposed films. Floor should be impervious to fluids and processing solutions and easy to clean. Walls and roof may be painted white or cream enamel such as paint can act as a good reflecting surface for safe light. It should be provision for running tap water and well ventilated but light proof. Entry to the dark room should be preferred through a double door with bolts inside avoid any accidental opening when processing is going on. It should neither be damp nor subjected to extremes of temperatures.

Dark room should have the following sections.
- Dry section.
- Wet section.
- Film hangers.
- Safe light.
- Lead boxes.

Dry section
- Dry bench is for loading and unloading of the films into the cassettes.
- Dry bench should have enough space to open the largest cassette and preferably of 3'x 2' dimensions. The height of the bench should be of 3' so that anyone can able to work comfortably.
- There should be provision of cupboards under the bench top to store the cassettes, timer, film marking devices etc.
- Safe light should be provided to illuminate the area.
- A waste paper basket should be available.

Wet section

- Wet bench is for processing of the film. Usual set up is to install a thermostatically controlled processing units or a sink (with provision of floating thermometer)

- China tiles should fix on the walls around processing and washing area.

- There should be a safe light in this section too.

- There should be provision for hanging towels in this area so that during processing hands should be washed and dried to load the cassette.

Film hangers

Types of film hangers: Channel type, Tension type, Clip type.

- In channel type of hangers, processing solutions may be retained in the channels which require careful cleaning for their maintenance.

- In clip type hangers, there is risk of clips scratching film during processing.

- A similar risk is also involved in tension type hangers.

- Different sizes of hangers are

  - 6 ½" x 8 ½"   ▪ 12" x 15"
  - 8" x 10"   ▪ 15" x 17"
  - 10" x 12"

Safe light

It is box containing a low watt (10 watt maximum) frosted bulb covered by a specific filter. One type of safe light is not suitable for all types of films.

Points should be considered

- Safe light should have correct filter

- It should be at least 3 feet away from the film

- Bulb in safe light must be of correct watt

- A film should not be left exposed to safe light

Films should be exposed to safe light only during loading or unloading of cassettes during processing

X-ray film processing

It is necessary to level the developer prior to beginning of processing of X-ray film. Select the correct film hanger. Thereafter switch on the safe light and switch off the white light before opening the cassette.

Processing solutions include

- ➤ Developer   ➤ Fixer
- ➤ Rinser   ➤ Replenisher for developer (washer).

Developer

Reduces silver halide crystals of the film to metallic silver which converts invisible image into visible image.

Composition of developer

Reducing agent: Hydroquinone or Metol

Activator: Sodium carbonate (softens and emulsion, alkaline medium, allows the reducing agent to act)

Restrainer: Potassium bromide (controls fogging activity of reducing agent)

Preservatives: Sodium sulphite (controls rapid oxidation)

Solvent: Water

Time: 4-5 minutes at 20 °C (never be kept for more than 3 months as its oxidation renders the solution unfit for use).

Rinser

To stop the action of developer solutions. Stop bath containing 128 ml of glacial acetic acid in 1 liter of water. Time: 10-30 sec at 27 °C.

Fixer

It is use to remove unexposed silver crystals on the film, neutralizing the action of developer, shrinks and hardens the film emulsion.

Composition of fixer

Fixing agent: Sodium thiosulphate or ammonium thiosulphate to remove unexposed crystals

Acidifier: Acetic acid or sulphuric acid (to neutralize the developer)

Hardener: Ammonium chloride or ammonium sulphide (shrinks and hardens the film emulsion)

Preservatives: Sodium sulphite (to maintain the chemical balance of fixer)

Solvent: Water

Time: 5-10 minutes

Film washing

Final washing removes the excess fixer and residual silver. It is done in large tank with the provision of running water. Washing time should be increased in case of prolonged fixing process. If washing is not proper, film gets discolored

Film processing steps

1. Check the level of the processing solutions, temperature and stir the solution.
2. Select correct size of the film hanger.
3. Switch on the safe light and off the white light.

4. Open cassette on the dry bench and take out the film by grasping the corner with thumb and index finger. Than film is fixed in a hanger.

5. Place the film in developer (4-5 min). Agitate the film for few second to remove air bubbles.

6. Lift the film out and allow the developer to drain and then view in the safelight for development of film (wet film viewing).

7. Rinse the film for 10-20 second.

8. Film transfer to fixer (double the time of developer-10 min)

9. Wash the film in running water.

10. Allow the film to dry.

Chapter 13

Intensifying Screens

The use of intensifying screens has three major benefits

1. Reduction of patient dose
2. Reduction of tube and generator loading and
3. Reduction of patient motion artifacts.

However, there is one disadvantage that is occasionally relevant to radiology which is that the image clarity is degraded in comparison with a directly exposed film.

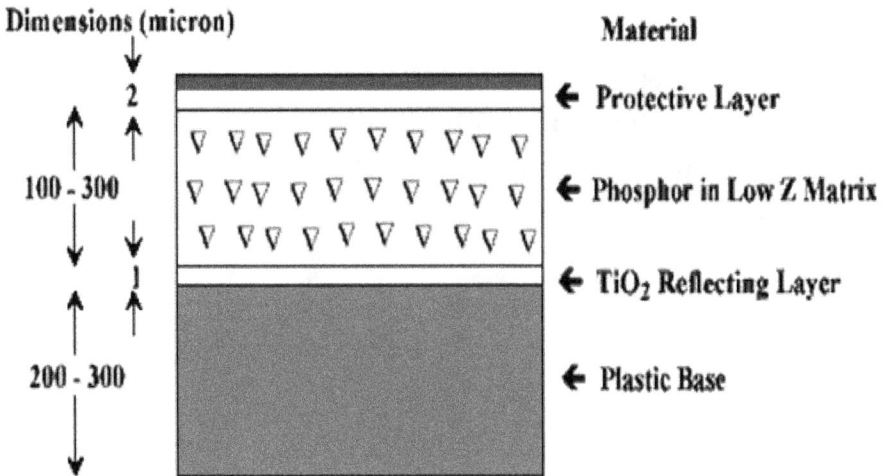

Figure 13.1: Cross-section of an Intensifying Screen. 1 micron = 1 mm.

A) **Base**: It provides mechanical support to active phosphor layer and is made of either high grade card board or polyster.

B) **Phosphor Layer:** Active layer of the screen and main function is to convert X-ray energy into visible light. The materials mostly used as phosphor in fluorescent screen are calcium tungstate, barium lead sulphate and zinc-cadmium sulphide.

C) **Reflecting Layer:** Thin reflecting layer is spread between the base and phosphor layer and made of shiny white substance such as titanium dioxide or magnesium oxide

D) **Protective Layer:** The thin transparent protective layer provides protection for the phosphor and can easily be cleaned. It consist of a cellulose compound

Rare earth screen

X-rays absorption efficiency of a pair of rare earth screen is 60 per cent *i.e* higher than that of a pair of tungstate screen (20-40 per cent). The conversion efficiency 20 per cent is much greater than the tungstate screen 5 per cent. Rare earth screen film combination has 12 time more fast speed than par speed tungstate screen film combination and thus X-ray exposure is reduce by 15-50 per cent. The increased absorption efficiency of the rare earth screens is due to improved absorption efficiency and not due to its increased thickness of phosphor layer. Phosphor use is activated gadolinium oxysulphide, terbium activated lanthanum oxysulphide, terbium activated yttriun oxysulphide and thulium activated lanthanum oxybromide.

Advantages

1. Exposure time is reduce and thus less motion unsharpnees.
2. Decreased patient's radiation dose.
3. Decreased scatter radiation.
4. Use of small focal sport is possible.
5. Increased tube life due to use of low mA.

Disadvantages

1. Cost of screen is high.
2. May require green sensitive X-ray films.
3. Exposure charts is more complex as screen response is kVp dependent.

Chapter 14

Radiographic Positioning in Animals

The objects for positioning the animal for radiography are,

(1) Greatest comfort of patient

(2) Restraint and immobilization of patient

(3) Accurate reproduction of part under examination in radiograph produced.

Nomenclature: In radiography terms, such as 'dorso-ventro', 'Ventro-dorso', 'Anterio-posterior' and 'Posterio-anterio' are used to denote the direction of the X-ray beam passing through the part under examination. The term lateral is used to describe radiograph in lateral plane. Sometimes the terms 'medio-lateral' or 'latero-medial' or oblique views are also used to denote the direction of the X-ray beam.

Number of Radiographs required: Since a radiograph is two-dimensional impression of three-dimensional structure, it is usually necessary to radiograph the part under examination at least in two planes in order to enable the veterinarian to visualize the part accurately.

Aids in positioning: These aids comprise things as non-radiopeque cushions, sand bags, blocks of wood, a compression band are employed to check movement of patient during radiography.

Identification of the film: The patient number or name and date of radiography and markers such as R (Right) or L (Left), number (0-9) must be placed on the cassette prior to radiography.

Restraint: Conscious and uncooperative animal has to be restrained satisfactorily in particular positions. Ferocious dogs, exited animals are difficult to handle during radiography. Tranquilization, Sedation or light general anaesthesia is essential for proper positioning of the patient.

Preparation of patient: Dog collars, harness or dirt on the coat of the animal if any are likely to come in between the part to be examined. Prior to radiographic examination elementary track should be emptied, by withholding food and if necessary by giving enema, when examination of G.I. tract has to be carried out.

Radiographic positioning:-

Small Animal

A. Forelimb

I. Scapula
i. Posterio-anterior view
ii. Lateral view

II. Shoulder joint
i. Posterio-anterior view
ii. Anterio-posterior view
iii. Lateral view

III. Humerus
i. Posterio-anterior view
ii. Lateral view

IV. Elbow joint
i. Anterio-posterior view
ii. Lateral view

B. Hindlimb

I. Pelvis
i. Ventro-dorsal view
ii. Lateral view

II. Hip joint
i. Ventrodorsal view
ii. Lateral view

III. Femur
i. Anterio-posterior view
ii. Lateral view

IV. Stifle joint

C. Skull
i. Dorso-ventral view
ii. Ventro-dorsal view
iii. Lateral view

i. Anterio-posterior view
ii. Lateral view

V. Radius and ulna
i. Anterio-posterior view
ii. Lateral view

VI. Carpus
i. Anterio-posterior view
ii. Lateral-oblique view
iii. Medial-oblique view
iv. Lateral view

VII. Metacarpus

VIII. Digits
i. Anterio-posterior view
ii. Lateral view
Posterio-anterior view
ii. Lateral view

V. Tibia and Fibula
i. Anterio-posterior view
ii. Lateral view

VI. Tarsus
i. Anterio-posterior view
ii. Lateral view

VII. Metatarsus
i. Anterio-posterior view
ii. Lateral view

D. Cranium
i. Anterio-posterior view
ii. Ventro-dorsal view

E. Nasal chamber

    i. Ventro-dorsal view

G. Teeth

    i. Dorso-ventral-intraoral view

    ii. Oblique view

I. Neck

    i. Lateral view

    ii. Ventro-dorsal view

II. Large Animal

A. Head

    i. Lateral view

    ii. Dorso-ventral view

    iii. Ventro-dorsal view

B. Neck

    i. Lateral view

    ii. Dorso-ventral view

    iii. Ventro-dorsal view

C. Forelimb-shoulder joint

    i. Anterio-posterior view

    ii. Posterio-anterior view

    iii. Oblique view

    iv. Lateral view

D. Elbow joint

    i. Anterio-posterior view

    ii. Lateral view

E. Radius and ulna

    i. Lateral view

F. Carpus

    i. Anterio-posterior view

G. Metacarpus

    i. Lateral view

    ii. Anterio-posterior view

H. Fetlock joint

    i. Anterio-posterior view

    ii. Lateral view

F. Tempero-mandibular joints

    i. Lateral view

    ii. Oblique view

H. Thorax

    i. Lateral view

    ii. Ventrodorsal view

    iii. Dorso-ventral view

J. Abdomen

    i. Lateral view

    ii. Dorso-ventral view

    iii. Ventro-dorsal view

I. Phalanx

    i. Lateral view

    ii. Anterio-posterior view

    iii. Oblique view

J. Hind Limb for young animals

    i. Lateral view

    ii. Ventro-dorsal view

K. Pelvis view

    i. Lateral view

    ii. Ventro-dorsal view

L. Femur

    i. Lateral view

    ii. Anterio-posterior view

M. Stifle joint

    i. Lateral view

    ii. Anterio-posterior view

N. Tibia

    i. Lateral view

    ii. Anterio-posterior view

O. Tarsus

    i. Anterio-posterior view

    ii. Lateral view

P. Abdomen

    i. Rumen-lateral view

    ii. Reticulum-lateral and dorsal reticulopathy

Chapter 15

Interpretation of X-Ray Film

Radiographs should be viewed on a good evenly light viewing box in a semi darkened room. Dorso-ventral chest, ventro-dorsal abdomen or skull is viewed with a right side of the film facing the viewers left side. Lateral view radiographs are viewed by placing it facing left. Radiographs of extremities are viewed with lateral aspect on left side of the viewer. Do not view the radiograph at a too close range, particularly a radiograph of the abdomen and thorax. Often an abnormality may be missed if the examiners eyes are too close to the viewer. For study of fine bone structures, examine the part with eyes close to the radiograph. Spot light should be used for examination of large animal radiography.

Interpretation

The aim of Veterinary radiography is to obtain radiographs of good technical quality from which radiographic diagnosis can be made. The field of diagnostic radiography based interpretation or reading of the radiographic details of the part.

The steps that list be followed before interpretation of radiograph is as under.

Step-1: A complete and detailed knowledge of animal and medical history must be obtained for proper evaluation of radiograph.

Step-2: Physical examination must be earned out. The purpose of radiography is to confirm a clinical diagnosis; detailed physical examination is necessary first to establish the reasons of radiographs and second to determine the part or parts of animal to be radiographically examined.

Step-3: Correct radiographic procedure is extremely important. A radiograph changes a three-dimensional subject into a two-dimensional flat plane. For this reason it becomes necessary to make at least two views at 90 degrees to each other. Although the best radiograph, interpretation can be a challenge. Loss of quality decreases the diagnostic usefulness of the radiograph. Therefore there should not be loss of radiographic details, density and contrast either during processing or after processing of the X-ray film.

Special radiographic techniques such as use of contrast media, non-routine positioning greatly increases the usefulness of a radiograph.

Interpretation of radiographs

Radiographic diagnosis has two steps.

1) Location of lesion: Determining whether or not an abnormal structure exists.

2) Classification of lesions: Making a definitive or differential diagnosis.

   Basic radiographic signs of pathology are alterations:-

   a) Sized)   Density

   b) Architecture   e) Contour

   c) Position   e) Function of the region or organ

Classification of lesions

The lesions can be classified as under,

   (1) Developmental   (4) Metabolic

   (2) Traumatic   (5) Infectious

   (3) Neoplastic   (6) Degenerative

Chapter 16

Radiographic Quality

A good diagnostic radiograph is one in which have excellent details, correct density and the proper scale of contrast. The proper use of various radiographic exposure factors kVp, mA, time and FFD must be employed.

Detail

Detail is the degree of definition or sharpness of an object on a radiograph. Good detail is the true reproductions of an object.

The factors affecting the detail are:

- Shorter Focal Spot film distance
- Closeness of the object to the film.
- Use of intensifying screen.
- Movement of either the patient, cassette on movement of the machine.
- Screens, film contrast.
- Over exposure or under exposure.
- Focal spot size.
- Any condition fogging the film will bring out loss of detail.

Density

It is the degree of blackness on the process film. It is determined by the amount of light absorbed by an exposed film and is a measure of the degree of blackness of the film. Radiographic density is affected by the subject density which the weight per unit volume of different body constituents. The density of the radiograph varies directly with milliamperage, provided all other factors remain constant. Higher milliamperage produces more density and lower milliamperage produces less density. Radiographic density varies directly with exposure time.

Contrast

It is the difference in the various densities on a processed radiograph. Contrast is the difference between blacks, grays and whites. There can be long scale contrast and short scale contrast. Radiographic contrast varies inversely with the kilovoltage. The lower the kV produces a radiograph with a "short scale of contrast". Secondary radiation and scattered radiations causes lack of contrast. Improper development of film and use of warm developer cause lack of contrast. To get good radiograph in veterinary patients the following technique should be followed.

- Fastest exposure time possible (To prevent movement blur)
- Higher kvp
- Constant distance
- Constant milliamperage

Chapter 17

Radiographic Lesion

Bones /Joints

General radiographic signs of a bone disease

- ❖ Altered contour of the bone.
- ❖ Altered size of bone.
- ❖ Altered density of bone.
- ❖ Altered trabecular pattern.

General radiographic signs of a joint disease

- ❖ Widening or narrowing of the joint space.
- ❖ Altered contour of joint surfaces.
- ❖ Increased of tissue density around the joint.

1. Fracture

A break in the continuity of bone depicted by a line of radioleucency, when the fragments are distracted and by a line of radiodensity when the fragments are superimposed or impacted.

2. Acute osteomyelitis

In adult

- ❖ No bony change but increased soft tissue density is evident.
- ❖ Loss of demarcation between fascia and muscle bundles.

In young animal

- ❖ Young animals with acute metaphyseal osteomyelitis may show some irregular radiolucent zones in the metaphysis.

3. Chronic osteomyelitis

- ❖ Extensive increased soft tissue density.
- ❖ Speculated and radially oriented periosteal new bone growth is seen along the outer margins of main bony cortex.
- ❖ Cortical thinning.
- ❖ Sequestrum in the area.
- ❖ Involucrum (Bonylysis seen as an area of radioleucency in the radiodence bony image)
- ❖ Fungal osteomyelitis mimic radiographic signs of bone neoplacia

4. Hip dislocation

- ❖ Abnormal increase in intra-articular space.
- ❖ Abnormal angulation of bone in the area of joint.

5. Hip dysplacia

- ❖ Flattening of femoral head.
- ❖ Shallow acetabulum.
- ❖ Poor conformation of femoral head into the acetabulum.
- ❖ Increased joint space.
- ❖ Subluxation (Partial displacement) of femoral head from the acetabulum.
- ❖ Centre of femoral head is medial to cranial edge of acetabulum – No abnormality.
- ❖ Centre of femoral head is directly caudal to cranial edge of acetabulum- Hip dysplacia is moderate.
- ❖ Centre of femoral head is dislocated further caudal to cranial edge of acetabulum – Hip dysplacia is severe.
- ❖ Osteophytes in advanced cases.

6. Rickets

- ❖ Wide irregular growth plates in long bones.
- ❖ Cupping of adjacent metaphysis.
- ❖ Reduced bony density.
- ❖ Cortical thinning.
- ❖ Bowed diaphysis.

7. Osteosarcoma

- ❖ Illdefined increase or decrease in the bone density with the production of new bone growth around the affected area.
- ❖ Sunburst appearance of new bone growth.

Abdomen

1. Gastric torsion

❖ Greatly distended gas filled organ occupying major portion of the anterior abdomen.

2. Pyloric obstruction

❖ Enlargement of the stomach

❖ Accumulation of fluids/material (accumulation of barium) in pyloric area.

3. Intussusception

❖ Sausage shaped mass with increased density.

❖ Thin layer of gas outlining the layers of intussusception.

❖ Barium enema- "coiled watch spring" pattern.

4. Hydronephrosis

❖ Large mass with a smooth outline in the anterior abdomen filled with fluids with appearance of homogenous density.

5. Kidney calculi

❖ Small irregular radio dense areas roughly central to the kidney outline.

6. Cystic calculi

❖ Radiopaque cystic calculi easily visualized.

7. Prostate enlargement

❖ Relatively dense mass just anterior and ventral to the pelvic brim in the portion normally occupied by the bladder which is displaced anterior-ventrally.

8. Metritis and pyometra

❖ Slight thickening and enlargement of uterus may be uniformly tubular or sacculated and displacement of the colon.

Esophagus

1. Esophageal achalasia

❖ Distended organ occupying the upper half of the chest in the lateral view.

❖ Dorso-ventral view distended organ projecting beyond the shadow of the spine.

2. Esophageal foreign body

❖ Thickening of the esophageal wall.

❖ Increased density from that of the surrounding tissues.

Skull

1. Fracture

❖ Occult fractures associated with soft tissue swelling.

❖ Discontinuity of bony structures.

2. Temporo-mandibular luxation

❖ Displacement of mandibular condyles away from the post glenoid process.

3. Infectious disease

❖ Infectious process of the alveolus appears as a zone of lucency.

❖ Local sclerosis.

❖ Sinusitis - radiographic density in the sinus.

4. Neoplasia

Osteoma- Rounded sclerotic smooth mass of bone arising from the cortex with active periosteal response.

Osteogenic sarcoma- Proliferating bony lesion with the evidence of bone invasion and active new bone proliferation at its margins and sclerosis "Sunburst appearance".

5. Bone cyst

❖ Characterized by well-demarcated radiolucent areas within the bone and may be associated with cortical thinning as from bone expansion.

6. Nutritional osteodystrophy

❖ It represents deficiencies in mineralization of normally formed osteoid.

❖ Lamina dura is not seen due to improper osteoid formation.

❖ Advanced cases have evidence of bony demineralization.

7. Mandibular perostitis

❖ Sclerosis and active new bone production at the tympanic bulla or the mandibular sinus.

Chapter 18

Contrast Radiography

The main aim of contrast radiography is to obtain a good radiograph with enhanced visualization and demarcation from the tissue itself or its surrounding structure. It is done with help of some contrast media (Positive or negative).

Contrast techniques

1. Positive Contrast

Barium or water soluble iodide or oily and viscous preparation may be used as positive contrast media. Micro pulverized barium suspension 2 to 5 ml/kg body weight is administered slowly into the buccal cavity. Stomach tube may also be used to administer the contrast agent directly into the stomach.

2. Negative Contrast

Room air is given by a stomach tube 6 to 12 ml/kg body weight or carbonated beverage 30 to 60 ml may be given. This study is useful to locate radiolucent foreign body.

3. Double Contrast

Either air through a stomach tube or a carbonated beverage may be given before or after the use of barium. Water soluble iodine compound 7 ml/kg body weight by using stomach tube should be used when perforation of the esophagus, stomach or intestine.

Contrast technique of different organ

1. Dacrocystorhinography

Dacrocystorhinography is the contrast radiographic study of the nasolacrimal duct. This is indicated in cases suspected of partial or complete obstruction, atresia, inflammation, deviation or distortion of the nasolacrimal duct. Quick radiographic exposures are required if water soluble agents are used because of their rapid drainage.

2. Sialography

Contrast radiographic study of the salivary glands and duct is called sialography.

3. Bronchography

Bronchography is the radiographic visualization of the bronchial tree after infusing oily contrast media into the airways. Bronchography should be done cautiously in patients with cardiopulmonary diseases. Only one lung should be investigated at a time.

4. Esophagraphy (Barium swallow)

The technique is used to evaluate both structural and functional status of esophagus after introduction of a positive contrast media. Esophagraphy is indicated to diagnose case of esophageal obstruction, stenosis, diverticulum and mucosal diseases.

5. Reticulography

To diagnose cases of diaphragmatic hernia in buffaloes and cattle by feeding barium sulphate suspension to the animal.

6. Barium series

The procedure is indicated to evaluate structural and functional status of gastrointestinal tract. The technique should be avoided if rupture of the stomach or intestines is suspected. It is routinely used in small animals but is of limited value in large ruminants.

7. Peritoneography

The technique is indicated to visualize outlines of various abdominal organs and to locate a suspected abdominal mass. In this negative contrast agent (pneumoperitoneography) or a combination of a negative and a positive contrast agent (double contrast peritoneography) is used.

8. Renal angiography

To visualize renal vascular architecture and also helps to assess renal cortex to medulla ratio.

9. Myelography

It is a contrast radiographic examination of the spinal cord and emerging spinal roots after injecting the contrast material into the subarchnoid space. It is indicated to diagnose intervertebral disc protrusion, intraspinal lesions, vertebral canal haemorrhage and spinal cord oedema. It should not be used in cases of meningitis, myelitis and myelomalacia.

10. Arteriography

The technique refers to the contrast radiographic examination of arterial system of an area. It is indicated to study the arterial pattern in normal subjects and also to diagnose arterial occlusion.

11. Fasciagraphy

It is a contrast radiographic study of tendons and associated structures. The technique can be used to diagnose adhesion, calcification and rupture of tendons and muscle.

12. Intravenous pyelography (excretory urography)

Intravenous pylography (IVP) is a contrast radiographic examination of the kidneys and ureters after introduction of positive contrast medium. Apart from being an aid to diagnose abnormalities of urinary tract, the technique also serves as a rough index to kidney function. It should never be used in severely dehydrated patients because of risk of fatal anuria.

13. Urethrography

The technique is indicated to diagnose abnormalities of urethra in male such as urethral obstruction, stenosis and fistula.

14. Cystography

It refers to the contrast radiographic examination of urinary bladder and is indicated to diagnose structural abnormalities and diseases of bladder such as cystoliths, carcinomas and rupture of bladder.

15. Barium enema

It is used to outline the colon and rectum in the case of intra or extra luminal obstruction. Deep sedation or general anaesthesia is required eliminating straining. A 15-20 per cent (W/V) concentration of barium 20 to 30 ml/kg body weight is slowly administered through a cuffed rectal catheter by using syringe.

Chapter 19

Ultrasonography

Ultrasound is defined as sound waves of frequencies greater than audible to human ear. In ultrasonography a sound wave travels in a pulse and when it is reflected back it becomes an echo and this pulse echo principle is used for ultrasound image. Ultrasound transducers have piezoelectric crystals. When this crystal is stimulated electrically, it changes its shape and produces sound waves of a particular frequency which is determined by times of the crystal expands and contracts per minute. As the transducer is placed in close contact with the body surface through a coupling medium, it undergoes continuous modifications which occur through three processes: absorption, reflection and scattering. Absorption process forms the basis for therapeutic ultrasound. The reflection process forms basis of ultrasound scanning where echoes produced from different tissues are converted by piezoelectric effect into electrical signals and displayed on to an oscilloscope screen. Scattering occurs when the beam encounters an interface that is irregular and smaller than the sound beam. Conversion of echoes into electrical signals and subsequent visuals is known as echo quantification.

Uses

1. Scanning of liver, kidney, urinary bladder, spleen, uterus, ovaries, teat and udder for any type of deformity.
2. Pregnancy diagnosis in animals

Scanning procedure

A) Patient Preparation

In highly temperament animals, tranquillizer/sedative may be advocated before examination. Overnight fasting of the patient is advised if possible. Laxative may be given on the previous day to clear bowel of faeces and gas.

Patient should be prepared by clipping, shaving and cleaning the hair and skin. Ultrasound jelly should place in area of interest liberally to keep good contact of the transducer and having minimum attenuation of the sound beam.

B) Patient Positioning

Position of the patient is important to get acoustic window for proper image. Scanning may be performed by placing the animal on dorsal, lateral or in standing position depending upon the organ to be scanned and availability of good acoustic window. Full urinary bladder acts as good acoustic window for scanning of pelvic organs.

C) Image interpretation

Terminology used for image interpretation is

1. Hyperechoic/echogenic: - It is bright echoes and appears as a white in the screen.

2. Hypoechoic: - It appears as a grey images or dark screen.

3. Anechoic: - When in the screen no appear any echoes and it appears as black.

4. Acoustic enhancement: - A normal bright area immediately deep to fluid.

5. Artifacts.

a) **Acoustic shadow:** It is reflection or attenuation of sound beam at an acoustic surface. Here, bright image with no visible structure beneath a soft tissue/fluid filled cavity is seen due to presence of bone, minerals or gas inside the cavity. This is useful for detection of cystic, renal and biliary calculi.

b) **Reverberation:** It is the largest source of positive artifact. When sound beam is returned back to the transducer, a portion of beam is absorbed by crystals which form electrical impulse and image is shown in the screen. Rest portion of beam is reflected back in to the patient and to the transducer.

c) **Mirror image:** Occur at high reflection.

d) **Comet tail:** It is caused by a highly reflective interface most commonly the air fluid interface.

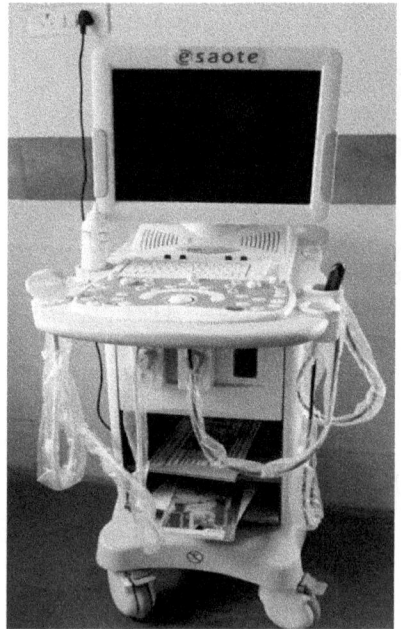

Figure 19.1: Ultrasonography machine

UNIT II

Chapter 20

Examination of Oral Cavity

Gross abnormalities and occlusal evaluation can be done under conscious examination, but for definitive oral examination requires general anaesthesia.

Examination

Examination should be gentle and limited to visual inspection and some digital palpation. Occlusion should be evaluated in the conscious animal. The mouth is first examined gently holding the jaws closed and retracting the lips to look at the soft tissues and buccal aspects of the teeth. This is the optimal time to evaluate occlusion, premolar alignment, distal premolar/molar occlusion, individual teeth positioning. Finally open animal's mouth. Most of the animals allow at least a cursory inspection of the oral cavity, once the jaws have been opened. The mucous membranes of the oral cavity and teeth should be examined. In addition to these, conscious examination involves the palpation of face, temporo-mandibular joint, salivary glands and lymph nodes.

Types of mouth gags are used for examination of oral cavity.

1. Varnell's mouth gag.
2. Bayer's mouth gag for horses and cattle.
3. Bayer's mouth gag for dog.
4. Hausmann's gag.
5. Carrez's gag.
6. Jogger's mouth gag for horses.
7. Buttler mouth gag.
8. Drink water's mouth gag.

Exploration of Mouth

Horse and cattle

- Put a halter around the horse.
- Pass the left hand into the interdental space on the right side.
- Catch the tongue gently and firmly.
- Draw the tongue outside the mouth.
- Pass the thumb of the right hand inside the left cheek at the commissure of the cheek.
- Draw the left cheek outwards to expose the gums and teeth.
- Reverse the hand to examine the other side in the same way.

Dog

- Place the right hand under the throat between the fingers and thumb.
- Grasp the lower jaw.
- Pass the left hand gradually down the face and grasp the upper jaw with fingers and thumb.
- Release the hold with right hand.
- Depress the lower jaw by placing the thumb of the right hand on the inner aspect of the incisor teeth.

Cat

Separate the jaws by means of two index fingers applied to the upper and lower incisor.

Examination under General Anaesthesia

- ➢ The oropharynx should be examined prior is endotracheal intubation. Examine the soft palate, glossal arch, tonsillary crypts and tonsils.
- ➢ Lips and cheeks: Examine the musculocutaneous junction, frenula and salivary papilla.
- ➢ Oral mucous membranes: Examine the alveolar mucosa, mucogingival line, attached and free gingival lines.
- ➢ Floor of the mouth and tongue: Sublingual caruncle, lingual frenulum, lingual salivary gland and tongue papillae.
- ➢ Teeth: Examine the dentition (primary/permanent/mixed) missing teeth/ supernumerary teeth, abnormalities in size, shape, position, angulation, wear patterns, pathological conditions like cavities, tooth fracture and enamel hypoplasia.

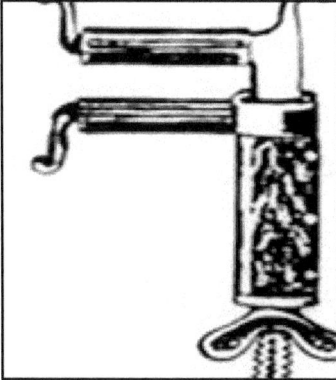

1. Varnell's mouth gag

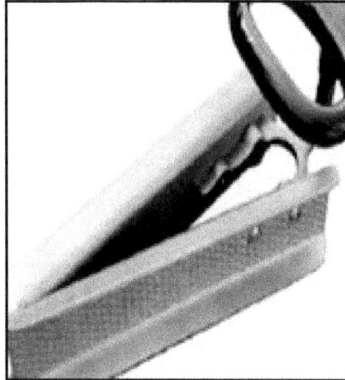

2. Bayer's mouth gag for horse and cattle

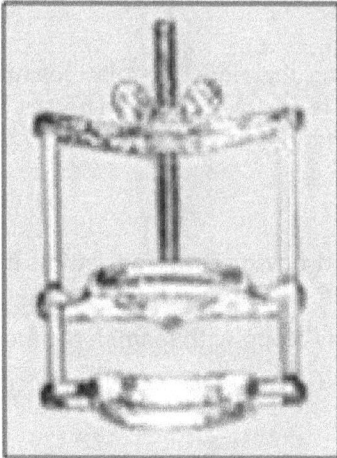

3. Buttler's mouth gag

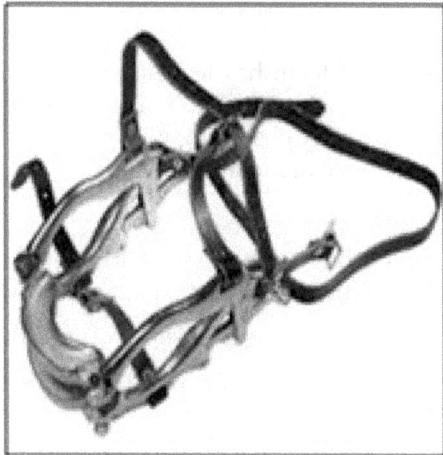

4. Hausmann's mouth gag (closed)

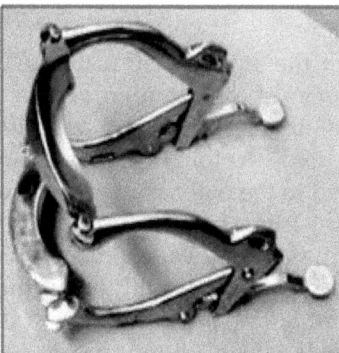

5. Hausmann's mouth gag (open)

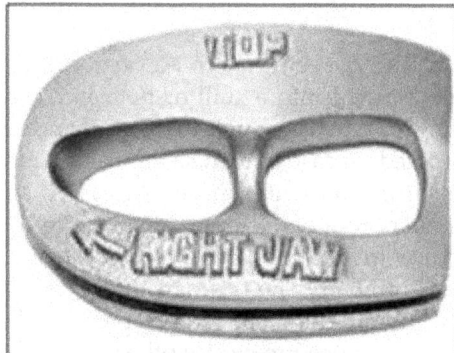

6. Drink water mouth gag

Figure 20.1: Different mouth gags

Chapter 21

Rasping of Tooth

Rasping of teeth has to be carried out when there are irregularities of wear and tear of teeth. Irregularities of wear in molar teeth are common in horses. Sharp teeth are generally observing with the outer border of the upper and inner border of the lower row of molar teeth.

Symptoms

a) Quidding of the food: Partially chewed hay or corn and letting it drop from the mouth saturated with saliva.

b) Salivation: This is observed continuously along with foam in the mouth.

c) Imperfect grinding which is recognized by absence of normal grinding sound.

d) Holding the head to one side when chewing.

e) Food collecting between the teeth and the cheeks.

Procedure

Rasping of teeth has to be carried out with the animal well restrained. The horse is backed into a stall or held into the corner of the room; in case of cattle securing in a travis is helpful. The mouth needs to be opened and a mouth gag can be used. In case of cattle an assistant gently holds the tongue out of the mouth through the interdental space. The rasp is applied to the outer border of the upper and inner border of the lower molar teeth. The rasp is run freely from one extremity of the row to another, taking care not injury to the soft tissues. There are different patterns of rasps. The ordinary hand rasp may be large or small to suit the size of the animal. The teeth require periodical attention for this condition. The rasp should not be used to excess otherwise; it will make the teeth too smooth to have a grinding effect. Once rasping is over appropriate treatment for lesions in the mouth must be carried out. Application of borax glycerine on the gums will help to soothe the painful lesions.

Chapter 22

Trephining of Sinus in Large Animals

Bovine

Trephining of the frontal sinus

Indications

It can be performed for empyema, tumour, cyst, depressed fractures and removal of isolated fragments of bone and exploratory purpose.

Anaesthesia and Control

Local infiltration. The animal may be controlled in the standing or cast position.

Anatomy

The frontal sinus in the bovine may be outlined by,

Lower limit: Line connecting the inner canthi of the eyes.

Upper limit: Frontal crest and into horn cores.

Lateral limit: Frontal ridge (temporal or lateral ridge of frontal bone).

The frontal sinus of each side is separated by the median septum. Each sinus is divided into a number of incomplete compartments by ridges of bone. The sinuses drain into the nasal fossa directly through cribriform plate of the ethmoids (while in horse it drains through maxillary sinus).

Blood supply

The frontal branch of the external ophthalmic artery enters the supraorbital canal and ramifies chiefly in the frontal sinus.

Sites

1. To obtain complete drainage from the post-orbital diverticulum, about 1 to 1½ inch above the upper border of orbit and medial and close to the temporal ridge.

2. Above a horizontal line connecting the supraorbital processes and at a point between the midline and the supraorbital fissure which accommodates the frontal vein and artery. This site is not satisfactory due to the risk of puncturing the cranium.

3. Below the base of the horn.

4. Amputation of horn or trephining into horn core will also open the frontal sinus.

Technique

Make an outline of the circumference of the trephine by direct pressure on skin with the trephine. Make a circulate incision of a slightly larger diameter and undermine the skin. Scrape and remove the facia to expose the bone. If the frontalis muscle is thick and interfering with the approach it has to be cut and retracted. Fix the centre of the trephine head on the bone and by applying pressure, work in a to and fro semi-rotary fashion till the thickness of the plate of bone is removed. Keeping a gap at lower level for drainage of fluid approximates the skin edges.

Trephining of the maxillary sinus

Indications

For removal of a diseased upper molar tooth, chiefly the fourth and for exploratory purpose in empyema.

Anaesthesia and Control

Local infiltration, standing or cast position.

Anatomy

In the bovine the maxillary sinus is not divided into superior and inferior compartments. It communicates with the middle nasal meatus by a slit-like opening. The fourth and fifth cheek teeth are rooted in the sinus. The third cheek tooth is partly rooted in it.

Site

Above the facial tuberosity and a variable point behind it according to the tooth to be removed.

Technique

Similar to trephining of frontal sinus.

Equine

Surgical Anatomy

Frontal sinus

> Frontal sinus in horse is not as extensive as that of cattle. The median septum divides right and left sinuses.

> The frontal sinus is divided into frontal and turbinate parts and further sub divided in small compartments by number of bony plates. Each compartment communicates with each other by small openings.

> The frontal bone lines the roof of sinus which extends anteriorly with anterior margin of orbit and caudally to temporal condyles and laterally to the foot of the supraorbital process.

> The turbinate part is located in the posterior part of the dorsal turbinate bone covered by nasal and lachrymal bones.

> The turbinate part is separated from the nasal cavity by a thin tissue of dorsal turbinate bone.

> The frontal and maxillary sinuses communicate with each other through a large fronto-maxillary opening, which is situated ventral to the osseous canal and medial wall of the orbit.

> The frontal sinus has no direct communication with the nasal cavity.

Maxillary sinus

> Maxillary sinus is the largest sinus in horse. It is divided into anterior and posterior compartments by an oblique septum.

> It is formed by the superior maxillary, lacrymal, malar and posterior turbinate bones.

> The boundaries of this sinus are:

• Medially -Maxilla, ventral turbinate and lateral mass of the ethmoid bone.

• Posteriorly -The border extends upto transverse plane in front of root of the supraorbital process.

• Anteriorly- Line drawn from the anterior end of the facial crest to the infraorbital foramen parallel to the facial crest.

• Ventrally- Alveolar part of maxilla.

> The sinus is irregular and four cheek teeth project into it.

> The sinus communicates with frontal sinus and nasal cavity.

Site

Frontal sinus

Locate the anterior border of sinus with the help of thumb and index finger passing backward along the nasal bones. The point where thumb and finger begin to diverge from each other forms the anterior limit of the sinus. The site of operation is about 3-4 cm posterior to this point and about 1-2 cm lateral to the median line.

Maxillary sinus

The anterior maxillary sinus is trephined at above 2.5-3.0 cm posterior and 2 cm medial to the lower end of the zygomatic ridge.

Posterior maxillary sinus is trephined about 2 cm medial to the lower end of the zygomatic ridge.

Surgical technique

Frontal sinus

Same as bovine.

Maxillary sinus

1. Enter the maxillary sinus in the posterior compartment at the proposed site.

2. Irrigate with 1:1000 potassium permanganate solution.

3. For entering the anterior chamber, another trephine opening is made.

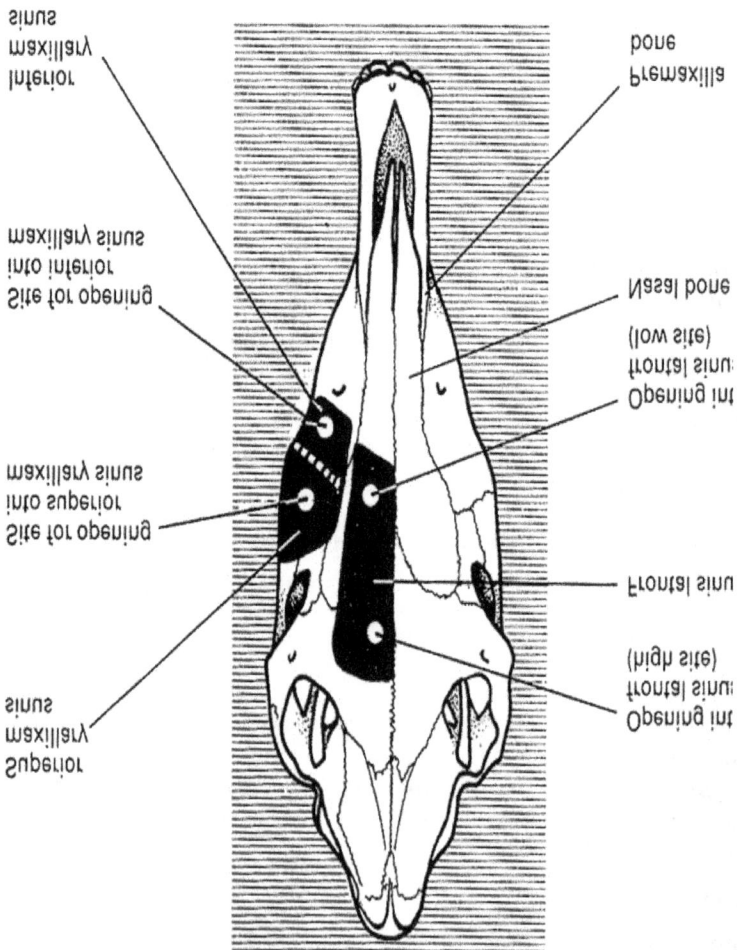

Figure 22.1: Frontal view of the horse skull showing the high and low sites for trephining the frontal sinus, sites for trephining the superior and inferior maxillary sinuses.

Chapter 23

Amputation of Horn

Indications

1. It is performed in the conditions of irreparable injury.
2. Malignant diseases.
3. For making better management and easy control.

Anaesthesia and Control

Cornual nerve block is performed. Animal restraint in the standing or in the recumbent position.

Anatomy

The horn core is a part of the frontal bone.

Blood and nerve supply

Cornual is a branch of superficial temporal artery and corresponding veins. Cornual nerve, it is a branch of the lachrymal, which is a branch of the ophthalmic branch of the trigeminal (fifth cranial) nerve (CLOT).

Sites

1. Below the base of horn after "flapping" the skin.
2. Any level below the seat of damage.

Techniques

Method-1: The flap method: The amputation is carried out through the frontal bone below the base of horn after flapping the skin forwards and backwards in two halves by a long elliptical incision around the base of horn, extending from the nuchal crest to the frontal ridge, long enough to expose the site of amputation. The bleeding is controlled with ligating the vessels and the operation is completed by suturing the skin flaps in apposition by interrupted sutures, after trimming the flaps as required.

Method-2: Amputation at the desired level is carried out by the direct method using a saw. Bleeding is controlled by thermocautery.

Method-3: Amputation is done with using dehorning shears. This is feasible only if the horn is small.

Method - 4: Disbudding in calves. Indications

1. For safe restraining the animals.

2. Avoid risk to other animals and the farmer.

3. To increase the aesthetic value of the animal.

4. For safety of transport.

Optimum age: Preferably five to fifteen days old.

Procedure

The calf should be sedated with xylazine and local infiltration at the site. The equipment consist a circular tip which can be applied around the horn bud, and having a long handle with necessary electrical connections. It usually operates on 220 volts AC. The connection is plugged to the electrical supply for five minutes till the circular tip gets sufficiently hot. The current supply is then cut off and the circular tip is applied slowly and steadily encircling the horn bud, for about half a minute, thereby destroying the horny tissue. The electric dehorner is also provided with different accessories which can be fixed on to the tip for other purposes of thermocauterization, like point firing, pin point firing, branding.

Method-5: Destruction of the horn buds by applying potassium hydroxide sticks, so that the horn growth is completely suppressed. It can be done in young calves when they are five to ten days old.

Chapter 24

Ligation of Stenson's Duct

Indication

In case of persistent salivary fistula, ligation of the duct brings about pressure atrophy of the gland.

Anaesthesia and Control

Local infiltration anaesthesia and controlled in the standing or recumbent state.

Anatomy

The stenson's duct arises from the ventro-medial aspect of the gland and proceeds along with ventral and anterior border of the masseter muscle to open into the buccal cavity in level with the fifth upper cheek tooth.

Sites

1. **Anterior or Distal site:** Immediately in front of the anterior border of the masseter muscle and about ½ to 1 inch above the inferior border of the horizontal ramus of the mandible where the duct can be palpated.

2. **Posterior or Proximal site:** In the Viborg's triangle which is outlined by the posterior border of the vertical ramus in front, tendon of sternomaxillaris above and the submaxillary vein below.

Surgical technique

A ½ to 1 inch long skin incision made along the course of the duct is made at the mention site. The head is held well extended if the posterior site is chosen. Identification of the duct is easy after cutting through the subcutaneous fascia, by its pink colour and anatomical relationship. Injury associated vessels is avoided. After exposing the duct ligated it with a broad, non-absorbable suture material like silk. Suture the skin wound by interrupted apposition sutures.

Chapter 25

Otoscopy and Othaematoma

Otosopic observations of ear canal

Normal structures

- ➤ Light pink, smooth and contains minimal exudates.
- ➤ Ear canal opening diameter varies with breed.
- ➤ Tuft of hairs present in front of the tympanic membrane can be viewed with otoscope.

Abnormal appearance

- ➤ Erythema, stenosis, proliferation, ulceration and foreign body.
- ➤ Presence, consistency and color of any exudates.
- ➤ Moderate to severe hyperplasia.
- ➤ Dilation of apocrine glands (Cocker spaniels).

Othaematoma (Aural haematoma)

It is condition when blood is accumulated in the layer of conchal cartilage and the skin of ear.

Anaesthesia and Control

General anaesthesia is preferable in dogs, and lateral recumbency with affected ear above.

Anatomy

The conchal cartilage is adhered with skin on its internal and external aspects. The blood collection (haematoma) between the skin and cartilage may be either on the internal or external aspect of the concha.

Techniques

Many treatments have been advocated for haematoma, varying from simple aspiration to complicated surgical techniques.

Method-1: Aspiration may be effective when haematoma is very small. It is repeated as often as necessary (2 to 3 times weekly) until serum no longer accumulates. A protective bandage should be applied with pressure exerted over the area of haematoma. If the haematoma is extensive, however this method is time consuming and likely to fail. Therefore surgical intervention is needed.

Method-2: There are many surgical techniques for operating ear flap haematoma. Best results are obtained if surgery is performed 10 to 14 days after formation of the haematoma. Many surgical incisions like longitudinal, 'S' shape and criss cross for removal of an aural haematoma have been practiced. 'S' shape incision is generally preferred since it covers more surface area of the aural haematoma. The haematoma is incised over its entire length longitudinally after plugging the external auditory meatus. The blood and blood clots are mobbed. A series of mattress sutures are applied through the edges passing through the thickness of the concha. Drainage is helped by removing an elliptical piece of skin from either edge of the incision. The ear flap is then turned over the head and a bandage is applied with pressure.

Method-3: It is similar as method-2 except that instead of mattress sutures. Flat buttons or coins with holes are kept on either side of the earflap through which the sutures are passed. The advantages are: (i) The apposition between the surfaces is more intimate (ii) The sutures are not likely to tear through the tissues and (iii) Bandage is not essential in this case.

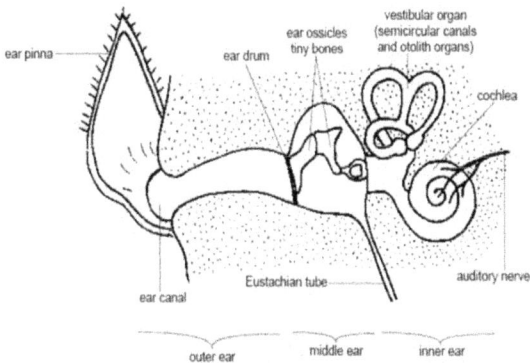

Figure 25.1: Anatomy of Ear

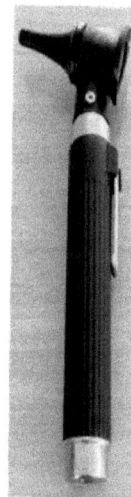

Figure 25.2: Otoscope

Chapter 26

Emergency Tracheotomy

Indications

1. Threatened respiratory failure (obstruction of the upper respiratory tract like oedema of the larynx, oedema of the upper lip and nostrils).

2. In prolapse of rectum to prevent persistent straining.

3. In persistent epistaxis.

Anaesthesia

Local infiltration.

Anatomy

The trachea is a cartilaginous tube has a number of incomplete annular cartilages, covered by sterno-thyro-hyoid muscles on the ventral face.

Blood and Nerve supply

The blood supply to the trachea is chiefly derived from branches of the common carotid arteries. The veins go mainly to the jugular veins. The nerve supply is from the vago-sympathetic trunk.

Site

It is 1 to 2 inches longitudinally along the ventral aspect of neck, preferably at the junction of its upper and middle third.

Surgical technique

An incision about 2 inches long is made through the skin and sub cutis on the mid-ventral line of the neck. After retracting the two sterno-thyro-hyoideus muscles, an incision is made between two tracheal rings. Insert the knife into the interannular ligament and partly cut through the upper ring. With the help of forceps grasp the cartilage through incision and continue the incision on lower ring, thereby excising a semicircular piece from the two adjoining rings. After making the opening, introduce gently the tracheotomy tube. Then the tube is fixed to the sides of the skin incision by sutures.

Chapter 27

Esophagotomy

Indications

Esophageal obstruction, esophageal diverticulum.

Anaesthesia and Control

Bovine: Local anaesthesia, standing or recumbent state.

Canine: General anaesthesia, dorsal recumbent state in the case of cervical esophagotomy, lateral recumbency for thoracic approach.

Site

Bovine: On left side of the neck, along the superior border of jugular furrow and close to the level of obstruction.

Canine: Site is chosen according to the level of obstruction.

    a)   Cervical site: Mid ventral line of neck.

    b)   Thoracic approach.

    c)   If obstruction is close to the gastric end, it is relieved well through the gastrotomy.

Anatomy

Lateral to the esophagus is the carotid sheath containing the internal jugular vein, carotid artery and the common trunk of vagosympathetic nerve and the strnosuboccipitalis part of sternocephalicus muscle. Ventromedially the esophagus is related to the trachea and the recurrent laryngeal nerve. Dorsally the esophagus is related to the longus coli muscle.

Blood supply

It is through branches of the carotid and bronchoesophageal arteries for cervical segment and short branches of the gastric artery towards the terminal segment. Delicate branches from intercostals arteries in the thoracic segment run circumferentially to supply the esophagus.

Surgical technique

Bovine

An incision about 3-4 inches long is made along the superior border of jugular furrow cutting through the skin and cervical cutaneous fascia. The jugular vein is retracted after separating it from the broncheocephalicus muscle; to encounter the sternosuboccipitalis muscle which is pushed downwards; and by blunt dissection the esophagus lying adjacent to the trachea can be located. The esophagus is recognised by its characteristic pink colour. It is exposed by a tenaculum. The wall of the esophagus is incised longitudinally over the desired length to get into the lumen and the obstruction is relieved. The mucous membrane is sutured with interrupted apposition sutures with knots inside the lumen. Outer coat is sutured with interrupted or continuous apposition sutures with   to ½ inch spacing. The overlying muscles and skin are sutured only if conditions are suitable for primary healing.

Canine

Common points of obstruction in the dog are as under.

A. At the entrance of esophagus into the thorax.

B. Above the heart and, close to the diaphragm at the entrance of esophagus into stomach.

A. For cervical approach the procedure is as similar lines as in bovines except that the approach is through midventral line of the neck. The sternocephalicus and sternothyrohyodius muscles of either side are separated along midline to expose the trachea and esophagus.

B. For esophagotomy in thoracic region, thoracotomy operation is to be performed.

Chapter 28

Ophthalmoscopy and Tests for Blindness

An adequate physical and laboratory examination is essential to diagnose oculars lesions. Proper restraint of animals is very important before a thorough examination of the eye. Before examination the eyes should be thoroughly cleaned to remove any exudates present. The first inspection is done in daylight to observe any injuries, ocular discharges or abnormal movement of the eyeball. An ophthalmoscope can be used for this purpose. General examination of the eye is made for gross abnormality. Various reflexes of the eye are checked such as corneal, palpebral and nictitating. The cornea and the outer segment of the eye are examined. Measurement of intraocular pressure is also help to judge eye disease condition. Special examination can also be done apart from general examination such as ophthalmoscopy for examination of the fundic region. Corneal staining is used to ascertain the extent and depth of corneal ulceration if present.

Ophthalamoscopy

Method used for internal examination of the eye especially the examination of fundus and vitreous humour.

Indications

1. Lesions on the retina

2. Fundic degeneration

3. Congenital fundic anomalies

4. Examination of intraocular growths

5. Examination parts of cornea

Methods of Ophthalamoscopy

Direct ophthalamoscopy

Intraocular examination will be done directly with an ophthalmoscope. The image presented is in its original position. For examination of various parts of the eye the position of ophthalmoscope is kept as under:

0 to –3 → Fundus

0 to +5 → Vitreous humour

5 to 8 → Posterior of lens

8 to 12 → Anterior of lens

12 to 15 → Anterior chamber

15 to 20 → Anterior cornea

Procedure of examination

➢ Ophthalmoscopic examination should be done in a dark room.

➢ After effecting pharmacologic mydriasis, place the direct ophthalmoscope against examiner's eye and identify the patient's fundic reflection from a distance of approximately 50 to 75 cm. Most ocular fundi can be focused at 0 to -2 diopter.

➢ Use examiner's right eye to examine the patient's right eye and left eye to examine the left eye.

➢ Once examiner's identify the fundic reflection, move toward the patient to a point approximately 2 to 3 cm from the eye.

➢ Identify and examine the optic nerve first, followed by thorough examination of the remainder of the fundus in quadrants.

➢ Adjust the size of the circular spot of white light to the size of the pupil to minimize light reflection from the corneal surface.

➢ After examining the retina, the structures anterior to it are examined by changing the diopter dial from minus to plus values.

➢ Estimate the distance of the abnormalities in the retina by changing the dioptric power. Abnormalities viewed in minus diopters (red) are depressed and those viewed in plus diopters (green) are elevated from the retina.

Indirect ophthalamoscopy

In this method, the examination of internal eye is done with the help of a condensing lens kept between the eye and the ophthalmoscope. The image presented is small and inverted. It is better as it provides larger area for visualization and a stereoscopic image is presented. It is specifically used for diagnosis of fundic degeneration and retinal detachment.

Procedure of examination

• Ophthalamoscopic examination should be done in a dark room.

• Effective pharmacological mydriasis.

• Mount the binocular light source on the head and adjust the view through the eye piece.

• Hold open the eyelids and focus the light on the patient's eye.

- Position the lens 2 to 4 cm in front of the patient's cornea. The lens should be held with the thumb and forefinger, at one-arm-distance away from the light source. See that the more convex surface of the lens faces toward examiner's for the best image.

- Adjust the intensity of the light to avoid excessive illumination of the fundus.

- Correct the reflections from the surface of the handheld lens by slightly tilting the lens.

- Once examiner identifies the fundic reflection, he can visualize the opacities of the cornea, lens and vitreous in front of the reflection.

- Examine the fundus for the optic nerve, retinal vasculature and tapetal and non-tapetal fundus.

- Opacities will move as follows when the eye rotates in the dog and cat.

- Opacities anterior to the posterior lens nucleus will move in the same direction of eye rotation.

- Opacities posterior to the posterior lens nucleus will move in the direction opposite that of the eye rotation.

Tests for Blindness

Test for blindness is difficult in animals. True evaluation of pain, light and dark adaptation, field of vision and percentage of vision is practically impossible in animals. For subjective analysis of blindness in animals, good history is very important. Following tests can be performed in a dark room

1. Direct a light at the base of the nose from a distance of 2-3 feet to outline both pupils together. This is done for the evaluation of any difference in pupillary size.

2. Pupillary Light Reflex (PLR) – Use a bright light and shone it directly on to the eye and evaluate the response of the pupil to the light - This initiates the direct PLR. PLR will be clearly present, sluggish or absent. Swing the bright light to the contralateral eye within 3 seconds and observe the pupillary response. The initial observation will be the response of the pupil initiated by the light source on the first eye, and is called the indirect or consensual reaction. But as the light is maintained it initiates the direct reflex to the eye.

3. Menace response – Make a threatening, sudden movement near the eye, without causing any air current or without touching the eye lashes. This should elicit a blink reflex and is known as menace response. Make sure that the palpebral reflex is intact in animals negative for menace response.

4. Dazzle Reflex – Stimulate the retina by showing a very bright light against the eye. This should result in a bilateral narrowing of the palpebral fissure.

5. Visual placing – This is for animals which have a normal motor function and mental status. Hold the animal in space supporting the head and chest. Approach towards a table surface. As a normal response, the animal should extend and raise the legs anticipating standing on the table top.

6. Maze or Obstacle course test - Place several light weight obstacles in the path of the animal. Allow the animal to negotiate the space in dim and bright light. The ability of the dog to avoid the obstacles should be observed and graded.

7. Cotton ball test – Blind-fold one eye and swing a ball of cotton within the field of vision of the other eye. Assess the ability of the dog to follow the path of motion of the cotton ball by its eye and head movement.

8. Catoptrics test – This test is help for diagnosis of lens and corneal opacities. It is done in dark room. A lighted candle is used and holds it about 6 inches from the eye. In the normal eye three distinct images can be observed on the cornea, the anterior capsule of the lens and the posterior capsule of the lens, respectively. The first two images are erect and third one is invrted. The first image is large and bright where third image is small and least bright.

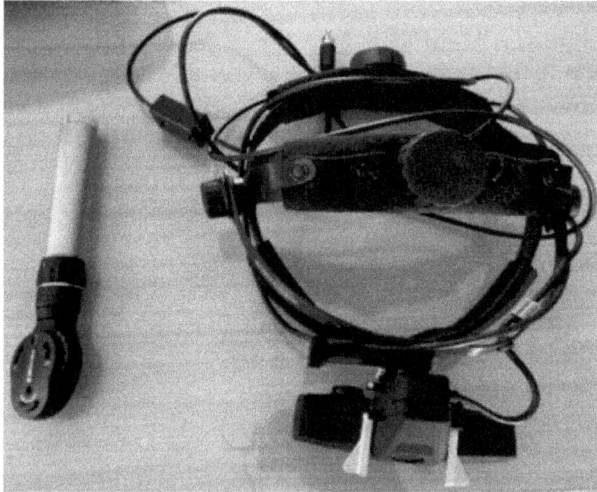

Figure 28.1: Ophthalmoscope- Direct and Indirect.

Chapter 29

Ectropion and Entropion

Surgical correction of ectropion

Indication

Outward deviation of the palpebral border.

Anaesthesia

Local infiltration.

Site

½ to 1 cm away from the free border of the eyelid.

Blood supply

Branches of the ophthalmic and facial arteries; the blood is drained by the corresponding veins.

Nerve supply

Sensory nerves are derived from the ophthalmic and maxillary branches of the fifth cranial nerve (trigeminal). The facial nerve supplies motor fibers to the muscles; occulomotor nerve supplies the levator muscle of the eyelid.

Surgical technique

A "V" shaped cutaneous incision is put to the affected border of the lid. The triangular flap of skin outlined is worked loose from its apex by cutting to effect correction of palpebral border. The gap thus created at the apex, is being closed with suturing the sides of the "V" shaped incision to form a "Y". It is usually the lower eyelid that is affected.

Surgical correction of entropion

Indications

Inward deviation of the palpebral border, trichiasis and districhiasis.

Anaesthesia

Block the facial nerve as it emerges on to the cheek. Below the temporo-orbital nerve as it comes out of supra-orbital foramen (Sensory to upper lid) or by field block.

Surgical technique

Take up a fold of skin parallel to and a short distance from the affected palpebral border by means of a special wide-jawed forceps or an ordinary dressing forceps, the depth of the fold being sufficient to bring the eyelid into its normal position by averting the border. Remove the fold of skin by cutting it with a sharp scissors and the wound is sutured by simple interrupted pattern using non-absorbable suture material.

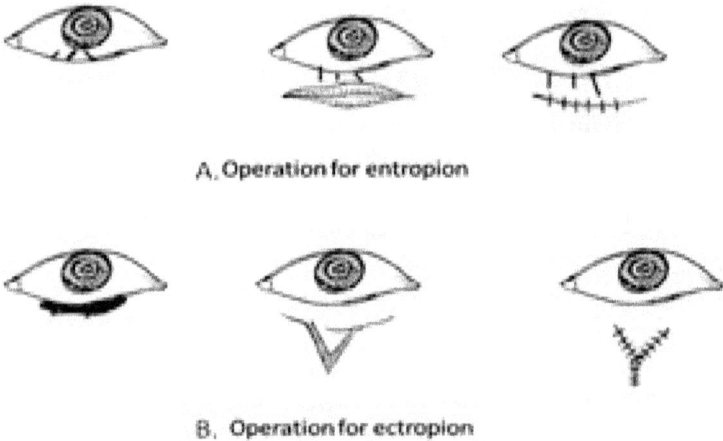

A. Operation for entropion

B. Operation for ectropion

Figure 29.1: Correction of ectropion and entropion

Chapter 30

Extirpation of Eyeball

Indications

Irreparable injury, orbital abscesses, malignant disease.

Anaesthesia and Control

General anaesthesia and controlled in lateral recumbent state.

Anatomy

The eyeball is situated in the bony cavity of the orbit formed by the frontal, lachrymal and malar bones. The conjunctiva lines the inner surface of eyelids and is then reflected on to the scleral surface (as palpebral and bulbar conjunctiva).

There are five straight and two oblique muscles of the eyeball.

1. Superior rectus.

2. Inferior rectus.

3. External rectus.

4. Internal rectus.

5. Posterior rectus.

6. Superior oblique.

7. Inferior oblique.

These muscles originate around the optic foramen and are inserted on the sclera behind the attachment of conjunctiva. The muscles are enclosed with a fibrous covering called as Tenon's capsule.

Blood supply

Blood supply is through external and internal ophthalmic arteries and veins. The external ophthalmic artery is a branch of the internal maxillary and the internal ophthalmic is a branch of the internal carotid artery. The orbital and periorbital veins form a venous plexus between the orbit and muscles of the eyeball. It communicates with the cavernous sinus and dorsal cerebral veins on the one side and frontal and facial veins on the other.

Nerve supply

Motor nerve supply: Superior oblique muscle by the fourth cranial or the trochlear nerve; Posterior and external rectus by the abducents or sixth cranial nerve; and the other muscles by the oculo-motor or third cranial.

Sensory supply: By the ophthalmic nerve and naso-cilliary nerves.

Techniques

Method -1: Enucleation of eye

The conjunctiva is held by forceps and is divided around the eyeball exposing the scleral insertions of the muscles of eyeball. These are divided one by one so that it will be possible to turn the eyeball and severe the rest of the attachments. The eyeball is removed and the orbit is plugged to arrest haemorrhage. If tarsorrhaphy is to be performed the edges of the lid are trimmed and sutured.

Method -2: Extirpation of eye

The palpebral borders of the eyelids are temporarily sutured together. An elliptical cutaneous incision enclosing this suture line is made without opening into the conjunctival sac. Retracting the skin edges, the eyeball along with its muscles is detached from the bony orbit by blunt dissection between the Tenon's capsule and bony orbit. After division of the attachments close to the base of the orbit and removal of the eyeball, the orbital cavity is packed with gauze to control bleeding. The skin edges are united by apposition sutures leaving a small gap at the inner commissar for removal of the gauze packing next day.

Canthotomy

A temporary canthotomy may be done during surgical operations of the eye when the lids are to be kept wide open or to facilitate the reposition of eyeball. It is done with incising the skin at the lateral canthus, which is sutured after the operation.

Chapter 31

Laparotomy

Indications

Laparotomy or opening of the abdomen may be undertaken for any of the following purposes:

1. Gastrotomy, Rumenotomy or Abomasotomy.
2. Enterotomy and Enterectomy.
3. Cystotomy.
4. Hysterotomy (Caesarean section) or Hysterectomy.
5. Ovarectomy (Spaying).
6. Spleenectomy.
7. Ventropexy (Rumenopexy, Omentopexy Abomasopexy, Cecopexy).
8. Exploratory laparotomy.
9. Repair of diaphragmatic hernia.

Anaesthesia

1. Field block by inverted "L".
2. Linear infiltration.
3. General anaesthesia.
4. Para-vertebral analgesia.

Control

1. Standing position for incisions through paralumber fossa.
2. Lateral recumbency for incisions in lower flank.
3. Dorsal recumbency for incisions through ventral abdominal wall.

Sites

Horse

1. Right flank incision: Base and apex of the caecum, ileocaecal junction, middle portion of the right ventral colon, right internal inguinal ring, right kidney and right ovary.

2. Left flank incision: Pelvic flexure of the colon, left ventral colon, spleen, left kidney, left internal inguinal ring and the left ovary.

3. Ventral approaches

a. Mid-line incision: Greater exposure of abdominal organs (for caesarian section, enterotomy in volvulus or torsion or incarceration).

b. Paramedian incision: Abdominal organs, better exposure of the bladder and uterus.

Cattle

1. Flank approaches

a. Upper left flank approach: Exploratory laparotomy, rumenotomy, left flank abomasopexy, repair of ruptured bladder and removal of mummified or macerated foetus.

b. Lower flank incision: Caesarian section in cows and buffaloes.

c. Upper Right flank approach: Exploratory laparotomy, abomasopexy, omentopexy, surgical correction of intestinal obstruction and caecal dilation.

d. Ventrolateral oblique incision: Caesarian section in cows and buffaloes.

2. Ventral approaches

a. Paramedian incision: Abomasopexy, caesarian section.

b. Median incision: Generally used to expose the non-pregnant genitalia in small ruminants for experimental purposes.

c. Post-xiphoid incision: Repair of diaphragmatic hernia.

Small animals

1. Right flank: Spaying.

2. Ventral Mid line approach: Gastro intestinal surgery and urogenital surgery.

Surgical techniques

1. **Flank site:** The skin is incised to the required length and avoiding division of lumbar spinal nerves, the incision is extended through the external, internal oblique abdominal muscles and the transverse abdominal muscle. The parietal peritoneum is picked up by tissue forceps and is first snipped open by scissors and this opening is then extended by scissors over finger

or grooved director introduced into it to prevent injury to viscera.

2. **Mid-line site:** The skin over the white line is incised to the length required. The sides of the white line are held by tissue forceps and lifted so that a small opening is made by cutting with scalpel between the forceps, through the white line and the adherent parietal peritoneum. A finger is introduced into the opening and the incision is extended to the required length by scissors over the protecting finger.

3. **Para-median site:** The incision is made parallel to the linea alba, through the skin, outer and inner coverings and belly of the rectus abdominis muscle and the parietal peritoneum.

4. **Para-rectus site (Lateral to the rectus muscles):** The skin, oblique abdominal muscles, aponeurotic sheath and the parietal peritoneum are to be incised. The incisions are being parallel to the rectus muscle.

5. **Para-costal site:** The incision is through the skin, oblique and transverse abdominal muscles and the parietal peritoneum parallel to the costochondral arch.

Laparotomy incision is closed in separate layer.

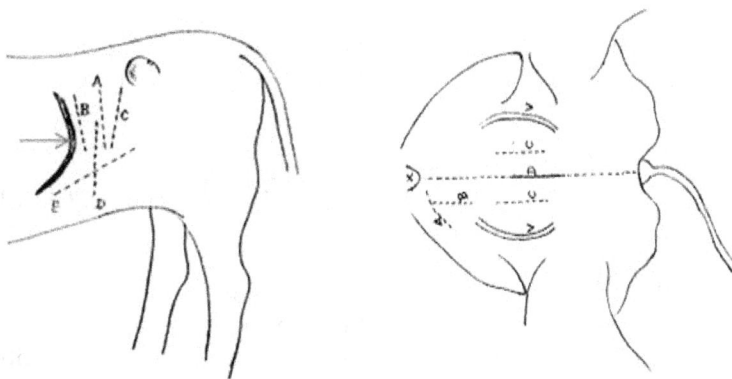

I. Flank region laparotmomy sites   II.   Ventral abdominal laparotomy sites

Arrow- Last rib

A) Mid upper incision	A) Post xiphoid
B) Caudal and paraller to last rib	B) Cranial paramedian
C) For urinary bladder approach	C) Caudal paramedian
D) Lower flank	D) Median line incision
E) Ventrolateral oblique incision	E) Subcutaneous vein

Figure 31.1: Laparotomy sites

Chapter 32

Thoracotomy

Thoracotomy in the bovine

Operation involves the cutting and removal of about 5 to 6 inches of the distal portion of the fifth rib of the left side.

Indications

To drain the pus and exudates collected in the pericardial cavity in certain cases of traumatic pericarditis. For remove any foreign body in the pericardium or close to it.

Site

Left side of the thorax over the fifth rib. The skin incision about 6 inches long is made from middle of the rib, downwards.

Anaesthesia and Control

Deep narcosis and local infiltration. The anaesthetic solution is injected along the anterior and posterior aspect of the rib and also deeply between the rib and the underlying parietal pleura. Amimal is controlled in lateral recumbency.

Surgical technique

The skin is incised (5 to 6 inches) over the rib. The underlying soft tissues are cut and retracted to expose the rib. A longitudinal incision is made on the middle of the rib to cut the periosteum. Then the periosteum is separated from the rib by using periosteal elevator or curved scissors. An obstetrical wire saw is introduced between the rib and inner periosteum, and then the rib is cut across at about 5 to 6 inches from its distal end. The cut end of the rib is held and is turned outwards to break it through the costochondral junction. The periosteum and parietal pleura are incised very carefully to avoid any sudden interference to the functioning of the lung. Sometimes the parietal pleura and pericardium may be adherent due to the local inflammatory process. If so, both these tissues may be incised together. In the bovine, the positive pressure ventilation is not required always, as the mediastinal septum in bovine is complete. After incising the pericardial sac, the fluid inside is removed and the cavity is irrigated with sterile normal saline and antibiotics. Incision of the pericardium is approximated with simple continuous sutures. The thoracotomy wound is sutured in three layers: the pleura and inner periosteum in first layer; the outer periosteum and thoracic muscles in second layer and skin in third layer.

Thoracotomy in the canine

Indications

1. Surgery of the thoracic portion of the esophagus.
2. Exploration of the thoracic viscera.
3. Thoracic approach for repair of diaphragmatic hernia.
4. Surgery of the lungs and heart.

Anaesthesia and Control

General anaesthesia; lateral recumbent state with the fore and hind limbs extended.

Site

Sixth or seventh intercostal space. Actual site depends on the purpose for which thoracotomy is performed.

Anatomy

The origin of the obliqus abdominis externus muscle is in close association with intercostal muscles, covering the lower half of the ribs from the fifth rib backwards. The latissimus dorsi muscle covers almost the upper half of the ribs. The posterior deep pectoral muscle covers the lower portions of the ribs, from the fifth rib forward.

Surgical technique

A cuffed endotracheal tube is introduced into the trachea up to the middle cervical level (Holding the tip of the tongue by a piece of gauze draws the tongue outwards, the epiglottis is depressed by a long forceps and the tube is introduced into the larynx and trachea). The free end of the tube is fixed with a tape to the upper jaw. The cuff of the tube now in the trachea, is inflated with air by a syringe and the inflating side tube is clamped. Connect the tube to a respiration pump or other device for positive pressure ventilation of the lungs. The skin over the intercostal space is incised parallel to the ribs. The serrated border of the muscle latissimus dorsi is first incised. A short incision is made through the middle ofthe intercostal muscles and parietal pleura, when the lung is in a deflated state. The incision is extended over finger introduced through it to protect the lungs. The rate and stroke volume of air inflated is adjusted according to the need. The ribs are retracted with self-retaining thoracic retractors and that side lung can be packed off with towels for mediastinal surgery. The thoracotomy wound is closed with interrupted sutures passed around the adjacent ribs. The last suture is tied when the lung inflated to its full capacity so that negative pressure would be restored as the lung deflates.

Another method of establishing negative pressure is by closing the intercostal incision with thin long rubber tube in the wound, the free end of which is kept below a water seal in a trough kept at a lower level, so that when the lung is inflated the air retained in the chest cavity is expelled through the tube whereas sucking air back is prevented by the water seal. The tube can then be removed. The layer of muscle is also brought into apposition by simple continuous sutures and skin incision is by horizontal mattress sutures.

Table 13.1: Surgical approaches for thoracotomy

Procedure	*Site of operation*
Thoracocentesis - Drainage of pericardial sac	5th to 7th Intercostal space
Pericardiectomy/Pericardiotomy	5th Intercostal space or 5th rib
Diaphragmatic herniorrhaphy	7th rib
Diaphragmatic abscess	6th or 7th rib
Pneumonectomy	4th to 5th rib
Transthoracic esophagotomy	8th rib

Chapter 33

Thoracocentesis and Abdomenocentesis

Thoracocentesis

Thoracocentesis is an invasive procedure to remove fluid or air from the pleural space for diagnostic or therapeutic purposes. A cannula or hollow needle is carefully introduced into the thorax, generally after administration of local anaesthesia.

Indications

1. For moist pleurisy condition to relieve respiratory distress.
2. Diagnostic purpose.

Anaesthesia and Control

Local anaesthesia; standing position

Site

Bovine

Due to complete mediastinal septa, thoracocentesis is done both sides to drainage fluid. In some case after proper diagnosis only affected side is process for thoracocentesis.

Left side

The sixth intercostal space and on a line with the point of the elbow close to the anterior border of the seventh rib.

Right side

The fifth intercostal space and on a line with the point of the elbow close to the anterior border of the sixth rib.

Canine

The seventh intercostal space on the left side and the sixth intercostal space on the right side above the level of the point of the elbow of the respective side.

Surgical technique

A trocar and canula about 6 inch long and 1/8 inch in diameter is used in the bovine and generally teat siphon is used in canine. The animal is secured in standing position and given local infiltration. The skin is punctured further behind the level of site chosen so that the puncture point does not coincide. The trocar is withdrawn to drain out the fluid.

In canine to prevent pneumothorax, a rubber tube, the free end of which is kept dipped in water, is attached to the needle; or the needle is attached to a syringe.

Abdominocentesis

Abdominocentesis is a procedure in which fluid is removed from the abdomen using a needle or trocar and canula assembly.

Indications

1. To drain abdominal fluid.
2. Ascites.
3. Diagnostic and therapeutic purpose.

Anaesthesia and Control

Local anaesthesia and standing or recumbent position.

Surgical Anatomy

The trocar and canula is to be directed through the skin, subcutis, oblique abdominal muscle, rectus abdominal muscle, the deep facia and parietal peritoneum to enter the peritoneal cavity.

Site

Lateral and behind the umbilicus

a) Left to the midline, approximately 3 to 4 cm and 5 to 7 cm cranial to the foramen, where the mammary vein enters the ventral body wall.

b) 10 cm cranial and 10 cm to the right of the umbilicus.

c) 5 to 10 cm caudal to the xiphisternum and 8 to 10 cm lateral (either right or left) of the midline.

Surgical technique

A small scalpel cut is made through the skin and a trocal-cannula assembly pushed carefully and slowly through the abdominal wall. The cannula will twitch when the peritoneum is punctured. Alternatively, an 18 gauge, 2 inch needle may be used, in which case local anaesthetic may not be required. A sample can be collected either by free flow or applying gentle suction with a syringe. If the initially chosen site does not yield fluid, the process may be repeated at another site a few centimeters caudally.

Chapter 34

Rumenotomy

Indications

Traumatic reticuloperitonitis (hardware disease), ruminal and reticular foreign bodies, frothy bloat, vagal indigestion, grain overload, toxin ingestion, chronic reoccurring bloat, creation of a permanent rumen fistula and exploratory rumenotomy

Site

Left flank in the paralumber fossa.

Anaesthesia and Control

Para vertebral nerve block or local infiltration analgesia (inverted "L" block or "T" block). Control in standing position.

Anatomy

The muscle fibers of the obliqus abdominis externus muscle run downward and backward; and that of obliqus abdominis internus muscle run downward and forward. The fibers of transverse abdominis are directed vertically.

Blood supply

The phrenico-abdominal and deep circumflex iliac vessels contribute the blood supply to the flank. The blood vascular channels of the rumen are located in the left and right longitudinal grooves and the anterior and posterior transverse grooves of it.

Nerve supply

Lumbar nerves: The flank is innervated by the thirteenth thoracic, first and second lumbar spinal nerves. In addition to this the third lumbar (cutaneous branch) supplies in front of the external angle of the ileum.

Surgical technique

A vertical incision about 6 to 8 inches long is made commencing about 2 inches below the level of the lumbar transverse process and 2 inches posterior to the last rib. The abdominal muscles and the parietal peritoneum are cut by a direct incision corresponding to the skin incision. The wound is kept retracted and the rumen wall is fixed by applying Vulsellum forceps with Weingart's frame. This is to prevent escape of rumen contents into peritoneal cavity. A short incision is made on the rumen and this is extended enough to permit easy access by hand into the rumen and reticulum. The incised ruminal wall is fixed to the Wingart's frame with rumenotomy hooks. The rumen contents are removed without contaminating the peritoneal cavity by proper packing. The reticulum can also be examined by stretching the hand through the wound in the rumen and the large rumeno-reticular passage and the esophageal groove and the opening of esophagus into the stomach are also palpable.

The incision on the rumen wall is closed with inversion sutures. Cushing and Lembert's sutures are used to close the rumen, commencing slightly above and extending a little below to the line of incision. The parietal peritoneum is closed with continuous sutures using No. 1 chromic catgut. The incised muscles are brought into apposition by simple continuous sutures. The skin incision is closed with horizontal mattress sutures or ordinary interrupted sutures.

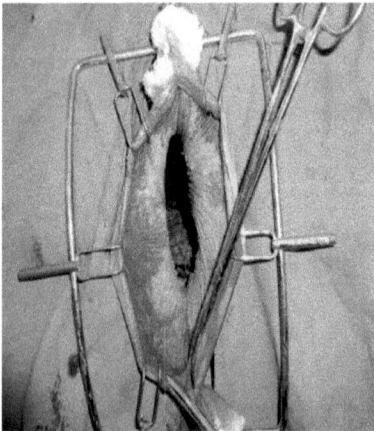

Figure 34.1: Intraoperative image of rumenotomy

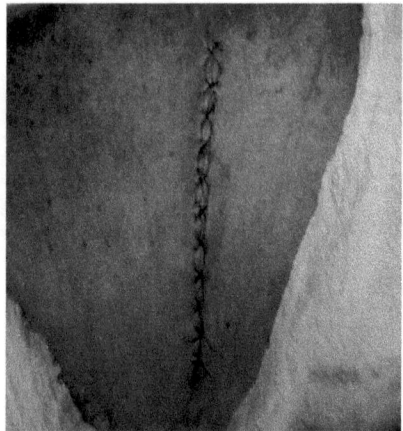

Figure 34.2: Closure of laparotomy wound

Chapter 35

Gastrotomy in Canine

Indications

For removal of foreign bodies from the stomach or from the gastric end of the esophagus. Gastric dilatation or gastric dilatation-volvulus (GDV).

Anaesthesia and Control

General anaesthesia and recumbent state.

Anatomy

The left fundic portion of the stomach lies under the vertebral ends of eleventh and twelfth ribs. The pyloric portion is situated towards the right of the median plane and lies almost ventral to the ninth intercostal space, between the xiphoid cartilage and costal arch of right side, in contact ventrally with the right central lobe of liver.

Blood supply

Branches of the celiac artery and veins drain into the portal vein.

Nerve supply

Vago- sympathetic nerve.

Sites

1. Mid-line incision between the xiphoid cartilage and the umbilicus.
2. Para costal incision on the left side in large and deep chested dog.

Surgical technique

The surgical site is prepared for operation. Perform laparotomy through mid-line incision. The stomach is exteriorized through the laparotomy wound and is packed off with surgical towels. The foreign body in the stomach wall is isolated in a pouch (the pouch may be clamped below with bowel clamps). An incision depending on the size of the foreign body is made along the length of the pouch or across it avoiding division of gastric vessels to the extent possible. The foreign body is extracted and the mucous membrane that pouch through the incision is trimmed level with the edges of the incision. The incision is closed by a set of Cushing sutures followed by continuous Lembert's suture over it. The surface of the stomach is cleaned with sterile saline solution and it is returned to the normal position after removing the packing towels. The laparotomy wound is closed.

Chapter 36

Intestinal Surgery

Enterotomy

Indications

Intestinal obstructions, foreign bodies.

Anaesthesia and Control

Dog: General anaesthesia and dorsal or lateral recumbent state.

Cattle: Field block or local infiltration and standing position.

Anatomy

The intestine is suspended by mesentery, which is a double fold of peritoneum encasing the bowel. The mesentery attached to it along one border only, conveys the blood vessels supplying the intestine, which are segment-wise or circumferential in distribution. The intestinal wall has a serous layer on the outside and a mucous lining facing the lumen with an intervening muscular coat.

Blood supply

Branches of celiac and anterior mesenteric arteries. Veins go to the portal vein.

Nerve supply

Vagus and sympathetic fibers from the celiac plexus.

Site

Mid ventral site or flank site.

Surgical technique

Perform laparotomy at the site chosen. The laparotomy wound is retracted and intestinal coils are examined to locate the foreign body by drawing the coils between the fingers. The affected segment of intestine is exteriorized and isolated by packing with surgical towels and is clamped before and behind with bowel clamps. A full thickness longitudinal incision is made on the free (anti-mesenteric) border in healthy tissue proximal to the obstruction. The obstruction is removed and the opening is closed by Cushing's sutures or by continuous Lembert's sutures. Size 3/0 medium chromic catgut with atraumatic needle is suitable for intestinal sutures. The towels are removed after cleaning the bowel surface with saline solution. The laparotomy wound is closed after returning the bowel into abdominal cavity.

Enterectomy and Enteroanastomosis

Indications

Intussusceptions with obstruction and adhesion, torsion, volvulus.

Surgical technique

Perform laparotomy. The segment affected is clamped at two points, before and behind using bowel forceps. The mesenteric vessels supplying the isolated segment are ligatured. The triangular piece of mesentery distal to the ligatures is torn towards the attached border of the segment and the bowel is divided close to the clamps and removed. The divided clamped ends are mopped clean and the stumps are closed with temporary continuous inversion sutures applied over the jaws of either clamp separately. The free ends of each thread are held and pulled as the forceps is withdrawn thereby closing each cut end of the intestine with this temporary suture. The closed ends are brought together and are united by Lembert's or Cushing's sutures all around. The temporary sutures are then drawn out and removed to establish patency of the ends after re-union. Patency is confirmed by feeling with the tips of fingers. The mesenteric tear is repaired. No part of the bowel wall should be left without blood supply. Return the bowel into the abdomen and close the laparotomy wound.

Different methods and techniques for enteroanastomosis:

Methods

1. End-to-end.
2. Oblique end-to-end.
3. Side-to-side.
4. End-to-side.
5. Telescoping.

Techniques

1. Parker-Kerr sutures: Parker-Kerr sutures are put as temporary stay sutures to close the cut ends until the anastomosing sutures are put.

2. Rankkins forceps: The Rankkins forceps with narrow jaws help to keep the cut ends closed until anastomosing sutures placed.

3. Ordinary hairpins can also be used in place of forceps.

4. Murphy button: Button has two pieces. These pieces are fitted into the cut ends by

means of purse-string sutures. Afterwards the two pieces of the buttons united. The button will be discarded in faeces after healing is completed.

5.   By using furnish clamp.

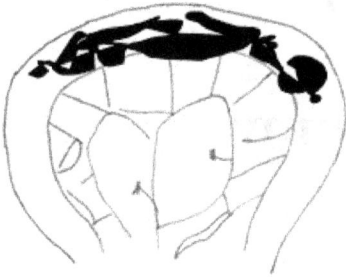

A. Affected intestinal part

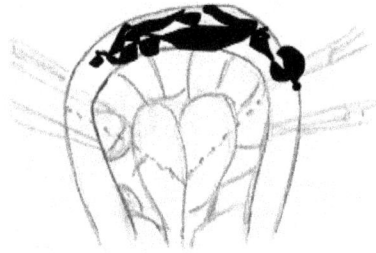

B. Hold affected part by intestinal clamp

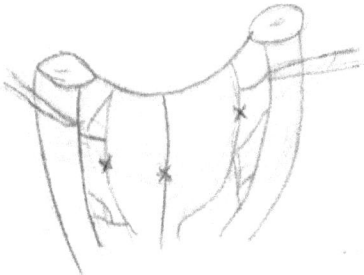

C. Resect affected part and ligation of mesenteric artery

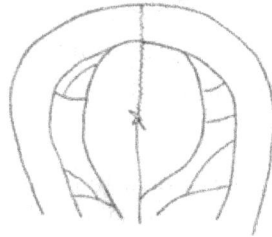

D. Enteroanastomosis

Figure 36.1: Technique of Enteroanastomosis

Chapter 37

Urethrotomy

Bovine

Indication

Urethral obstruction.

Anaesthesia and Control

Epidural anaesthesia and/or local infiltration. Standing or lateral recumbency.

Sites

1. Post-scrotal: To remove the urethral calculi from the sigmoid flexure. The incision is made on the mid-line about 3" behind the base of the scrotum.

2. Ischeal site: A 2" incision from the ischeal arch downwards along the mid-line.

Surgical techniques

Post Scrotal method

A 3" incision is made mid-line about 3" behind the scrotum, so as to cut the skin and subcutaneous tissue. The areolar tissue is dissected out to reveal the retractor penis muscles. These are separated and held retracted. The penile trunk is palpated and raised above the incision by hooking with fingers. The sigmoid flexure is exposed by giving traction to the penile trunk. The whole of the exposed penile trunk is palpated for the presence of calculi. The urethra is longitudinally cut into at the level of the obstruction. The calculus or calculi are removed to establish the patency of the canal. The penile trunk is replaced back and the skin incision is not sutured so that collection of urine in the surrounding tissue does not occur. Alternately, polyethylene catheter is passed through the urethra extending from the neck of the bladder to the tip of the prepuce where it is fixed with one or two sutures. Urethra is sutured over the catheter with interrupted sutures using fine silk or 3/0 chromic catgut. However; the skin incision is left open for drainage.

Postoperative care

The skin wound is dressed routinely. If the polyethylene tube has been passed then the bladder is daily flushed with sterile normal saline solution. The tube is removed on 10th or 12th postoperative day.

Ischeal site

A skin incision 2" long is made along the midline from the ischeal arch downwards. This exposes the bulbocavernosus muscle, which has to be divided to reach the corpus cavernosum urethrae. The incision on the body of the penis is made exactly on the mid-line so as to avoid damage to the branches of the internal pudic artery and exposes the urethra. A thick polyethylene tube is passed into the bladder by force through urethral opening. The tube is fixed to the skin by one or two sutures.

N.B.: This method is usually adopted in bull-calves to salvage them for slaughter.

Canine

Indications

Urethral obstruction, Urethral stenosis.

Anaesthesia and Control

General anaesthesia and controlled in dorsal recumbency. Operation is also possible in sedation and epidural anaesthesia or local infiltration.

Anatomy

Urethra is divided into three parts, the prostatic, membranous and the penile. The membranous portion located between prostate gland and the point where urethra dips into bulb of penis. After that urethra is a penile urethra, which extends up to the external opening. The whole urethra is enclosed within the corpus cavernosum urethrae, which is erectile and extremely vascular structure.

Blood supply

Urethral arteries.

Nerve supply

Pelvic plexus.

Site

Depending on location of calculus, incision is taken on midline over the urethra between os-penis and scrotum or behind scrotum at the level of ischial arch.

Surgical technique

Insert a suitable diameter gum elastic or polythene catheter. Hold the caudal end of the os-penis tense to skin with index finger and thumb. One to two centimeter incision is taken on midline skin; fascia and the fibers of the retractor penis muscles are separated longitudinally to expose the underlying corpus cavernosum urethrae. Incised the corpus cavernosum urethrae to expose the lumen. Remove the calculi. Press the bladder to remove calculi present in posterior part of urethra and suture the urethral mucosa and corpus spongiosum separately by simple continuous sutures using chrornic catgut size 3-0. Suture the subcutaneous tissue and skin.

Post-operative care: Dog should be observed for urination.

Chapter 38

Cystotomy

Bovine

Indications

1. Cystic calculi.
2. Cystic tumours.
3. Rupture of bladder

Anaesthesia and Control

Local infiltration after tranquillizing the animal. Standing or lateral recumbency.

Sites

Flank Site: Secure the animal in travis and right flank region is preferred.

Pre-pubic site: For small breed of cattle and in dorsal recumbency.

Surgical technique

Pre-pubic site: A 4" to 5" incision is taken on the skin starting from the pubic symphysis. The skin incision is on the lateral aspect of the penis in the male. The penis is deflected to one side and the linea alba is exposed. The abdomen is opened at the linea alba. The hand is introduced in the abdominal cavity; the bladder is identified and is brought to the incision. It is reflected on its neck and is isolated by packing from the abdominal cavity. A 2" incision is made on the dorsal surface of the bladder towards the neck to gain access into the bladder for necessary manipulations viz., removal of calculi, neoplasm or passing of a polyethylene tube into the urethra through the neck. The bladder incision is approximated with two layers of Lembert sutures. The opening of the linea alba is closed by interrupted or mattress sutures using No. 2 or 3 chromic catgut. The skin wound is approximated by mattress sutures using cotton thread.

Flank region: An 8" to 10" cm long incision was made in right flank for laparotomy. Introduce one hand for examine the bladder and correct the condition and catheterization. Blindly suturing of the bladder is carried out by continuous lock stick. Laparotomy wound is closed as per routine manner.

Postoperative care

If the tube has been passed, the bladder is daily flushed with sterile normal saline solution and an antibiotic solution is infused. The skin wound, is routinely dressed. The sutures are removed on 8th or 10th postoperative day.

Note: In the large animals the collapsed bladder cannot be brought to the incision. Hence, it has to be manipulated in situ.

Canine

Indications

1. Removal of cystic calculi.
2. Removal of neoplastic growth.

Site

1. In female, ventral midline about 4-5 cm. anterior to the pelvis.
2. In male, lateral to prepuce or below the penis through midline.

Anaesthesia and Control

General anaesthesia and hold the animal in dorsal recumbency.

Surgical technique

Urine is drained from the bladder if possible. Take incision as per sex, on skin and perform laparotomy. Take out the bladder through the incision. Pack the surgical wound with sterile gauze to prevent contamination of the peritoneal cavity. Then incision is made at the least vascular area on dorsal surface of the urinary bladder and calculi, if any, are removed. Then retrograde flush the proximal urethra to remove blood clots, tissue debris and small calculi which are loose in the lumen. After that the bladder wound is sutured with double row of Lembert sutures using chromic catgut No. 3-0 with atraumatic needle. Discard all contaminated instruments and close the laparotomy wound in usual manner.

Post-operative care

Remove urine frequently to minimize tension. Give anti-inflammatory and antibacterial agents. Give fluid therapy in dehydrated patients. Remove skin sutures after 8-10 days after operation or after complete healing.

Chapter 39

Vasectomy and Castration

Bovine

Vasectomy

Indications

1. To making a teaser bull.
2. Prevention of procreation.

Anaesthesia and Control

Local infliltration and control the animal in cast position.

Site

At anterior or posterior aspect of the neck of the scrotum, a little lateral to the median line.

Surgical technique

Take 5 cm incision through the skin and subcutaneous tissue, tunica vaginalis surrounding the cord. A pair of curved forceps is then introduced beneath the cord to elevate it and a long incision is made through tunic vaginalis communis in the area not covered by the cremaster muscle. Identify the vas deferens and clamp it with an artery forceps. Ligated the vas deferens on either side of the artery forceps and remove the piece after separating it from the attachment of the visceral layer of tunica vaginalis. The portion of vas deferens left back is not to be separated from their attachments to the visceral layer of tunica vaginalis to prevent the reunion of the cut ends. The scrotal incision is sutured with non-absorbable sutures. Operation on the other cord is done in the same manner.

Note: Examine the semen of teaser for viable sperms at every three months.

Caudectomy

Indication

To making a teaser bull.

Anaesthesia and Control

Local infiltration. In standing animal secured in travis or in lateral recumbency.

Site

Extreme end of the scrotum after holding the testicles taut.

Surgical technique

The lower testicle is held taut with one hand and a stab incision is put at the extreme end of the scrotum. The incision is bold enough so as to cut tunica vaginalis to expose the tail of the epididymis. The exposed epididymis is snipped with scissors. In the other method the body of the epididymis is ligated with 2/0 chromic catgut at two places about one centimeter apart and a piece of epididymis is removed between the ligatures. The open wound is dusted with antibiotic/ antiseptic powder. Sutures may or may not be taken. Similar procedure is followed on the other testicle.

Postoperative care: The wound is routinely dressed.

Castration- Closed Method

Indication

1. To prevent indiscriminate breeding.

2. For easy management and maintenance of working cattle.

Age: Three to six months.

Anaesthesia and Control

Local infiltration and lateral recumbency, casting the animal by castration method.

Site

The spermatic cord about 3 to 4 cm above the base of the scrotum.

Technique

The spermatic cord of the lower testicle is held taut against the scrotal skin. The blades of the Burdizzo's castrator are opened and the taut spermatic cord is taken in between the blades and crushed. The clamped blades crushing the spermatic cord are held in position for 30 seconds. The cord is once more crushed at a site 2 cm below the first site. The whole procedure is repeated on the other spermatic cord. Tincture iodine applied over the crushed marks. Precaution should be done that second time crushed clamp not on or the near scrotum.

Castration- Open Method

Indications

1. To prevent indiscriminate breeding.
2. For easy management and maintenance of working cattle.

Site

Posterio-lateral aspect of the scrotum.

Anaesthesia and Control

Spermatic nerve block. It is also advantageous to inject some amount of local anaesthetic into the testicular tissue. Standing with animal secured in a travis or in lateral recumbency, casting the animal by castration method.

Surgical technique

Open uncovered method

The scrotal skin together with the testicles is held taut from the base of the testicles. A bold incision so as to cut both the skin and the tunica vaginalis is taken on the posterio-lateral aspect of the testicles. The spermatic cord is exposed by giving traction to the testicles. The tunica vaginalis opening is extended with scissors so as to expose structures of the spermatic cord. The avascular part containing ductus deferens is separated from the vascular part. The avascular part is cut using emasculator. Alternately, it can be ligated using chromic catgut as high as possible and cut. The vascular part is ligated using chromic catgut as close to the abdomen as possible. The ligature is firmly anchored. The vascular bundle is then cut a little below the ligature. The bundle is released after ensuring that there are no bleeding points. The other testicle is also removed using the same procedure. Ablation of scrotal skin is carried out and the skin incision is sutured.

Open covered method

This method of castration is advisable if there is inguinal or scrotal hernia. The incision is limited to skin and subcutis, the testicle being exposed with its covering of tunica vaginalis tract. The spermatic cord is severed after ligaturing outside its covering.

Postoperative care: The wound is routinely dressed.

Equine

Castration

Indications

1. To make the horse docile.
2. Malignant diseases or irreparable injury.
3. Scrotal hernia.

Age: More than one year.

Anaesthesia and Control

General anaesthesia (TIVA or Inhalation) with spermatic nerve block in latero-dorsal recumbency.

Site

Ventral aspect of scrotum.

Surgical technique

The surgical technique is similar as in bovine described but precaution about aseptic surgery must be taken seriously to prevent complications of castration.

Canine

Castration

Indications

1. Prevention of breeding nuisance.
2. Neoplastic growths or crushing injuries affecting the testicle.
3. Enlarged prostate.
4. Perineal hernia.
5. To make dog more docile.

Anaesthesia and Control

General anaesthesia and dorsal recumbency with rear limbs gently abducted.

Sites

1. Prescrotal site: Midline in front of the scrotum.
2. Srotal site: Longitudinal incision on the ventral aspect of the scrotum, lateral and parallel to the median raphae on either side or longitudinal incision parallel to the median raphe.

Surgical technique

1. Prescrotal site: One testis is pushed forward and brought it under the skin, over the ventral aspect of sheath. An incision is taken over midline and testis is removed by pressing between thumb and forefinger. The cord is ligated and severed to remove the testis. Other testis is then removed through the same incision and skin wound is closed.

2. Srotal Site: Each testis is tensed against the skin of the scrotum and an incision is made anterio-posterioly parallel to the median raphe, cutting through the skin, dartos and tunica vaginalis. The testicle slips out through the wound. The spermatic cord is then separated into the anterior vascular bundle and the posterior bundle containing the vas deferens. The posterior bundle is divided with scissors and a self-legation is done with vascular bundle. The vascular bundle is then divided to remove the testis. The skin wound is left open. In longitudinal incision parallel to the median raphe on one side to remove that testicle and a second (through the same) on the mediastinum testes to remove the other testicle.

Chapter 40

Ovariohysterectomy and Caesarean Section in Bitch

Ovariohysterectomy

Indications

1. Elective sterilization.
2. Ovarian disease.
3. Uterine disease.
4. Behavioral problems.
5. Vaginal hyperplasia.
6. Prevention of mammary tumour.

Anaesthesia and Control

General anaesthesia and supine position or lateral recumbency

Site

1. Midline post-xiphoid.
2. On either flank or single long incision on right flank, parallel to the last rib, below the lumber transverse processes, at the level of the posterior lobe of the kidneys.

Surgical Anatomy

Ovaries lie close to the caudal pole of corresponding kidneys. Ovaries are covered with bursa and attached to the cranial ends of the uterine horn by the ovarian ligament. Ovaries are attached to the transverse fascia near the vertebral end of the last rib by suspensory ligament. Blood supply to the ovary is through ovarian artery and vein, which is a branch of aorta at 4th lumbar vertebra. The vein drains the cranial end of the horn of uterus and the artery anastomoses with the uterine artery. Uterine artery comes from the urogenital artery and enters the caudal part of the broad ligament at the plane of the cervix and lies close to the caudal part of the uterus. It gives 8-10 branches to the uterus and anastomoses with the ovarian artery.

Surgical technique

Take 2-3 cm long incision on the midline behind the umbilicus. Incise skin, subcutaneous tissue, linea alba, falciform ligament and peritoneum. Introduce an ovarectomy hook or index finger towards the left flank and uterine horn or broad ligament is withdrawn from abdomen. Apply three artery forceps, first close to ovary to hold severed vessels, middle one to hold stump from kidney and last, towards the kidney, in between above two artery forceps, to form groove for ligature. A double ligature with chromic catgut size 1-0 is placed on ovarian pedicle and the pedicle is cut between first and middle artery forceps. Haemorrhage is checked carefully. Similarly the right ovary is removed. The body of the uterus is then withdrawn from the abdomen and uterine vessels are ligated on each side and one ligature is applied to encompass the entire cervix. After that the broad ligament is cut then severe uterus just cranial to the ligatures. Check the uterine stump for haemorrhage and returned it into the abdomen. Close the abdominal incision in usual manner.

Caesarean Section

Indications

1.   Actual or potential dystocia.

2.   Fetal putrifaction.

3.   Elective C-section indicated in brachycephalic breeds and other animals with history of dystocia or those with pelvic fracture malunion.

Site

Midline post-xiphoid.

Anaesthesia and Control

General anaesthesia and in dorsal recumbency.

Surgical technique

Make a ventral midline incision from just cranial to umbilicus to near the pubis. Elevate the external rectus sheath before making a stab incision through the linea alba to prevent inadvertent laceration of the uterus. Exteriorize the gravid uterine horns by gently lifting rather than pulling out of the abdomen. Isolate the uterus from the remainder of the abdomen with sterile towels. Extend the incision with metzenbaum scissors. Empty each horn by gently squeezing cranial to each fetus to move it toward the incision. Then grasp and pull it from the uterus. Rupture the amniotic sac and clamp umbilical cord. Avoid contaminating the abdomen and surgical field with amniotic fluids. If the placenta has not separated gently pull it from the endometrium. Do not forcibly separate the placenta from the uterine wall. Palpate the pelvic canal and remove any fetus from this location. Close the uterine incision with 3-0 or 4-0 absorbable sutures using an appositional pattern in a double layer appositional closure. Lavage the surgical site. Inspect for uterine vessel avulsion and control haemorrhage. Cover the uterine incision with omentum. Appose the abdominal wall in three layers and suture the skin.

Post-operative care

1. Dress the wound with antibiotic ointments for 8-10 days. Give a course of antibiotic and pain killer injections.

2. Restrict the exercise for 10 -12 days.

3. Remove skin sutures after 8-10 days of operation or after complete healing.

Chapter 41

Amputation of Tail

Indications

1. Irreparable injury.
2. Tail gangrene.
3. Fracture of the coccygeal vertebrae.
4. Malignant disease.

Anaesthesia and Control

Epidural anaesthesia and animal secured in a travis in standing position.

Site

It is just proximal to the seat of injury or high up. If possible, sufficient length to cover the anus and vulva in female and anus in males should be left.

Surgical technique

A tourniquet is tied at the base of the tail. Two elliptical incisions are made, one on the dorsal and another on the ventral surfaces of the tail to raise two flaps of the skin. The base of the flap should correspond to the intervertebral space through which the disarticulation is to be effected. The tail is amputated by disarticulating at the joint. The tourniquet is loosened. The bleeding vessels are ligated. The skin flaps are approximated with mattress sutures with the knots on ventral surface. The tail is bandaged.

Post-operative care

The wound is routinely dressed and bandaged. The sutures are removed on 8th postoperative day.

Chapter 42

Ventral Hernia

A typical hernia has a hernial ring through which the contents have migrated and the hernial sac. A ventral hernia is caused by the migration of viscera through a tear in the abdominal wall. Umbilical hernia is situated in umbilical region and seen in generally young animal. Hernial sac in most cases is made up of peritoneum and skin. The sac may contents intestine, omentum, mesentery, abomasum or any part of gastrointestinal tract depending upon the location of ruptured muscles.

Anaesthesia and Control

Control the animal in dorso-oblique recumbency after sedation or tranquillisation. Infiltrate local anaesthetic at the site of incision and at the hernial ring.

Surgical technique

Take two elliptical incisions enclosing the sac. Expose the hernial ring and separate the patch of skin by blunt dissection. The peritoneal sac is then dissected carefully from the underlying tissue. Take care to avoid tearing of sac. Then the hernia contents are pushed into the peritoneal cavity. Close the hernial ring by over lapping sutures using chromic catgut size 3 or 4 or with umbilical tape in case of large ring. After that, take second layer of suture including fascia and suture the edges of ring with catgut size 2. Skin edges are apposed with interrupted sutures.

Post-operative care

1. Give systemic antibiotic for 5 - 7 days.

2. Animal is fed on reduced roughage diet for about 2 weeks after operation to minimize pressure on the site of incision.

3. Remove skin sutures after 10-14 days or after complete healing.

Chapter 43

Teat Surgery

Teat instruments

1. Teat plug: To retain medication inside the canal and also to plug the teat.
2. Teat bistoury: To enlarge the teat canal or to remove the growth inside the canal.
3. Tumour extractor: To remove the teat tumour or polyps from the canal.
4. Teat slitter: To cut the growth inside the teat canal is used for closed teat surgery.
5. Udder infusion tubes: For infusion of intra mammary medication.
6. Teat scissors: To trim the extra growth or to cut outside growth.

Teat canal obstructions

Interference in milk flow or difficulty in obtaining milk due to presence of

1. Lactolith (calculus).
2. Polyps.
3. Contracted sphincter of teat orifice.
4. Occlusion of teat orifice.
5. Membranous obstruction of teat canal.

Anaesthesia and Control

The anaesthesia either by local infiltration or injection of local anaesthetic though teat canal and control the animal in standing position.

Surgical Anatomy

Teat is derived from ectoderm. Teat orifice is the external opening of papillary duct (streak canal). Circular muscle surrounding the papillary duct prevents entry of foreign matter into the teat. Blood supply to mammary gland is the external pudendal arteries.

Surgical technique

A. **Lactolith:** It is freely moving calculi. It obstructs when it gets lodged at the orifice. If it is small, it will come out via orifice by milking. If it is large, crushed it by a mosquito or alligator forceps and remove it. If it is too hard and large, take a small cut on teat sphincter by "Lichty" teat knife or teat bistoury and remove the calculus.

B. **Polyps:** Polyps growth in canal is first localized then pass a teat tumour extractor into the teat canal and the polyps are removed.

C. **Contracted sphincter of teat orifice:** It is also called as hard milker. In such cases, insert "Lichty" teat knife or teat slitter or teat bistoury to enlarge the teat orifice. Then insert Larson teat tube to maintain the opening. Keep Larson teat tube for 5-7 days.

D. **Occlusion/absent of teat orifice:** Insert a 15-16 gauze hypodermic needle through the closed teat orifice until milk is flown out. A teat tube is inserted to maintain the teat orifice. Keep it for 5-7 days.

E. **Membranous obstruction of teat canal:** Instil 5 ml of 2 per cent lignocaine into teat canal. If obstruction is low in teat canal, ring block anaesthesia at the base of teat is sufficed. Insert a small teat bistoury up to fluctuating membrane and membrane is slit in three to four directions. Milk will flow down. Hudson spiral teat instrument is inserted and pulled to tear the membrane.

F. **Teat laceration:** It may not penetrate teat canal so milk flow will not allow from wound. After removing all foreign material and debridement, lacerated mass is closed. Two layer closer is done when laceration include muscular layer. The masculosa is sutured with simple continuous using polyglycolic acid suture or chromic catgut. The skin is sutured with interrupted pattern with cotton thread.

G. **Teat fistula:** It occurs due to penetration of the teat canal and fails to heal due continuous milk flow. If fistula is old and tissues around it have healed the tract should be excised. Elliptical incisions are made longitudinal to the teat on each side of opening and extended until entire tract is removed. The mucosa and masculosa are sutured with continuous pattern preferably with polyglycolic acid suture. The skin is sutured with interrupted pattern with cotton thread.

Post- operative Care

1. In case of teat sphincter surgery, teat cannula is necessary otherwise take out milk every after 15 min to 2 hours and then every 2 hours so as to prevent closure of orifice.

2. The animal should be completely and thoroughly milked daily and dressed with intra mammary antibiotic infusion, daily for 4 - 5 days.

3. Larson type teat tube is inserted to facilitate milking.

UNIT III

Chapter 44

Body Confirmation and Diagnosis of Lameness in Horse

Lameness

It is an indication of a structural or functional disorder in one or more limbs that is manifested during progression or in the standing position.

Synonym: Claudication

General Classification

❖ Supporting limb lameness

When the horse supports the weight on the foot. *e.g.* injury to bones, joints, collateral ligaments

❖ Swinging limb lameness

When the limb is in motion. *e.g.* pathologic changes involving joint capsules, muscles, tendons and tendon sheaths.

❖ Mixed lameness

When the limb is in motion and also supporting the weight.

❖ Complementary lameness

Pain in one limb cause uneven distribution of weight on another limb or limbs which can produce lameness in previously sound limb.

Examination of Horse for Conformation of Body

Forelimb and hind limb

To evaluate conformation the horse should be

❖ Observed from a distance and also closely

❖ Examine at rest and also in motion

❖ Examine for proper length, angulations from anterior, lateral and rear views

❖ Examine for various limb contacts

❖ Limb determine – Shape of feet, wear of feet , distribution of weight and flight of the feet

Faulty conformations of body

❖ Short backed horses and long backed horses

❖ Examination of lame limb suspected

❖ Examination of seat of lameness

Faulty conformations of forelimbs

❖ **Base Narrow:** The distance between the centre lines of feet at their placement on the ground is less than the distance between the centre lines of limbs at their origin.

❖ **Base wide:** Distance between the centre lines of the feet at their placement on the ground is greater than distance between the center lines of limbs at their origin in chest.

❖ **Toe in:** Toes point towards one another when viewed from front

❖ **Toe out:** Toes point away from one another

❖ **Base narrow–toe in**

❖ **Base narrow–toe out**

❖ **Base wide–Toe out**

❖ **Base wide–Toe in**

❖ **Plainting:** Placement of one forefoot directly in front of the other

❖ Posterior deviation of carpal joint

❖ Anterior deviation of carpal joint

❖ Medial deviation of carpal joint

❖ Lateral deviation of carpal joint

❖ **Open Knees:** It is irregular arrangement of carpal joint when viewed from side.

❖ Lateral deviation of metacarpal bone

❖ **Tied in knees:** When viewed from side flexor tendons appear to be too close to the cannon bone just below carpus.

❖ **Cut out under knees:** When viewed from side this condition causes a 'cut out' appearance just below carpus on anterior surface of cannon bone.

❖ **Standing under in front:** When viewed from side entire forelimb from the elbow down is placed to back of perpendicular and too far under the body.

❖ **Camped in front:** When viewed from side entire forelimb from body to ground is too far forward.

❖ Short upright pastern

❖ Long sloping pastern

❖ Long upright pastern

Faulty conformations of hind limbs

❖ **Base narrow**: It is distance between center lines of feet is less than distance between center lines at thigh region.

❖ **Base wide**: It is distance center lines of feet their placement on ground is greater than distance between center line at thigh region.

❖ Medial deviation of hock joints.

❖ Excessive angulation of hock joints

❖ Base narrow from fetlock down.

❖ Excessively straight legs/straight behind.

❖ Standing under behind – entire limb is placed too far forward / sickle hocks are present.

❖ Camped behind: Entire limb is placed far posteriorly.

Diagnosis of Lameness

❖ Anamnesis/ History
  • Duration of condition
  • Information about past incidence
  • Breed, sex, age, nutrition others
  • Past and immediate symptoms
  • History of shoeing.
  • Prevention, treatment and response

❖ Character of stride of limb
  • Phases of stride
  • Arc of foot flight
  • Path of foot in flight
  • Landing of foot

Visual examination

Proper thoroughly visual examination should require for detection of lameness.

❖ The swellings, enlargements, faulty conformations.
  ➢ Limb examination
    ▪ At rest
    ▪ During motion

- Landing of foot, placement of hoof, toe, heel
- Movement of head
- Arc of foot
- Swellings, faulty conformation
- Movement of all joints
- Various limb contacts

Examination by Palpation

Palpation should be start from the bottom of foot and make a complete examination of entire limb.

Forelimb Examination

> **Examination of bottom of foot**

Contraction of heels

Condition of frog

Condition of sole

Area of sensitively

Bruises, wounds, necrosis etc.

> **Hoof wall examination**

Excess dryness

Contraction, cracks

Wear and tear

> Coronary band - Presence of heat, wounds
> Lateral cartilages – Side bones
> Pastern area - Swellings, change in temperature, pulsation
> Fetlock Joint – Pain, osselets, distention, joint disease
> Cannon Bone – Splints, periostitis
> Suspensory ligament – Pain, scar, pupture, sprain
> Superficial and deep flexor tendons
> Carpus
> Soft tissues
> Elbow and shoulder joints :- Omarthritis, bicipital bursitis, cappled elbow etc

Hind limbs

> **Hock joint** – Bog spavin, bone spavin, occult spavin, curb, capped hock.
> **Stifle joint** - Gonitis

Upward fixation of patella

➢ Rupture of collateral or cruciate ligaments

➢ Hip Joint - Round liagament,

➢ Acetabular fracture, gait

➢ Pelvis - Fracture

➢ Tuber coxae, Tuber ischeii

➢ **Special examinations**

   Using hoof tester

   Local nerve blocks to determine site of lameness

   Radiography, Thermography, Ultrasonography

Chapter 45

Equine Shoeing

Shoeing is an art and a science. For farriers to do their best work, a proper area should be provided, and well-mannered (tractable) horses should be presented. There should be a place to tie horses safely at a height above the withers, and the area should be well lighted, uncluttered, and level. A concrete slab covered with a rubber mat is an ideal. Shade and shelter should be provided for summer as well as for winter work. Access to electrical outlets for power tools is essential.

The horse's movement should be evaluated at a walk and at a trot in a straight line so that the farrier can watch (from the front, rear, and side) the manner in which the horse picks up its hooves, moves them, and puts them down. From the side view, the hoof should land flat or slightly heel first but generally not toe first. From the front and rear view, the hooves should land flat. A hoof that does not land properly when it is time for a reset may indicate that the hoof was not correctly shoed in the first place, the hoof has grown out of balance since the last shoeing, the horse is compensating for pain, or the horse's conformation is such that the hoof does not land flat. The way a hoof lands differs with each gait and from forelimb to hind limb. Most horses require shoeing every 5 to 8 weeks, partly because the hoof wall at the toe grows faster than that at the heels, which causes the hoof to become imbalanced. After removing the old shoes, each hoof and shoe are examined for clues to wear patterns.

The hoof angle can be determined by using a hoof gauge, and the length of the untrimmed hoof can be measured with dividers or a ruler. The balance, shape, and symmetry of the hoof are assessed, and any tendencies to form flares or dishes are noted. Hoof symmetry and size are evaluated by comparing one hoof to the other.

Surgical shoeing

After the foot is properly trimmed and levelled, the desired surgical shoe of the correct size should be selected. The selected shoe must be fitted to the foot rather than the foot fitted with the shoe. While applying the shoe it must be centered accurately on the foot. Shoe may be applied hot or cold, but the hot method is preferred because, more accurate shaping can be done.

While employing surgical shoeing one has to think of two procedures, either an additional of obstruction or its removal. Addition of an obstruction will impede the rate and location of breakover, whereas, removal of an obstruction will enhance the rate and/or location of breakover.

A number of corrective or surgical shoes are available in such a way that the desired function of the foot can be achieved after surgical shoeing. Some of the important corrective shoes are as under.

1. Roller toe and square toe shoe

They are used to promote quick breakover by shortening the lever arm and sparing the work of flexor tendons. These shoes are indicated in the treatment of navicular disease, tendon problems and the problems of sesamoid ligament. They are also used to correct gait abnormalities viz., paddling, forging, winging etc. A roller toe shoe can also used in bone spavin and partial upward fixation of patella.

2. Bar shoe

Available types of bar shoe includes full bar, diamond bar, egg bar, V- bar, heart bar and half bar. These different types are used for following purpose.

1. To increase ground surface contact.
2. To distribute weight over a greater surface area.
3. To protect certain area of the foot.
4. To apply selective pressure.
5. To increase stability.

Full bar shoe is used in corns and navicular disease. Heart bar is used in laminitis. Egg bar and diamond bar shoe are used to reduce the concussion in condition like sheared heals. V-bar is used to protect frog region in condition like frog tenderness. Half bar is used to protect the affected side of the heel.

3. Heel clips, quarter clips and toe clips

These are used to reinforce the heel, quarter or toe region respectively, in cases of heel cracks, sand cracks, hoof cracks to secure the shoe to a weak walled hoof.

4. Trailer shoe

It is a shoe with one or both heel extended for corrective purposes. It is used in spavin, flexor tendon problems and problems with under run heels.

5. Shoe with elevated heels

It reduces the tension on deep digital flexor and tendon and decreases the concussion to the phalanges. It is used in navicular disease and the problems involving digital flexor tendon like tendosynovitis, tendinitis strains etc.

6. Wide web shoe

It increase surface area with the ground and protect the solar surface of the hoof. It is used in sole bruising, laminitis, etc.

7. Full roller motion shoe and pole shoe

They are used in condition like pyramidal disease, ring bone, side bones and forging.

8. Memphis bar shoe

This shoe possesses two bar across the branches on the ground surface and can be used in conditions like ring bone, side bone, flexor tendon problems and to correct gait abnormalities.

Chapter 46

Orthopaedic Care and Plaster of Paris Cast

The treatment of fracture includes: Four 'R'.

1. Recognition
2. Reduction
3. Retention
4. Rehabilitation

1. Recognition

Diagnose the fracture for suitable line of treatment.

2. Reduction

Holding the upper fragment of the bone and then moving the lower fragment into the correct position carry out the correction of the displaced fracture ends. For easy manipulation, administer general anaesthesia or a muscle relaxant. In case of limb, tie a rope round the pastern and give traction along the normal direction of the limb.

3. Retention

The reduced fragments are then retained in normal position till healing is complete, for that immobilization of the fractured fragments is necessary. This can be achieved by applying materials like a cloth bandage, plaster of paris and wooden splints, metal strips, metal sheets, etc.

Splints

Splints made of light metal or wooden sticks are applied after good padding with cotton wool over the affected part including both the nearest joints. The splints are kept in position by rolling a cotton bandage over it.

Rehabilitation

It will take months together for normal functioning of the limb.

General guidelines for bandage

- ➢ Animals often require chemical/physical restraint.
- ➢ Limbs and joints should be placed in nearly normal positions, unless elimination of weight bearing is required.
- ➢ Joints above and below to the injury need to be stabilized.
- ➢ Bandages and splints should be evaluated weekly for damage, soiling, or constriction of tissues.
- ➢ Post-splinting radiographs are useful in confirming adequacy of bone alignment.

Casting

Casts are a form of custom made external immobilization that lie in contact with the skin and are made to conform to the injured part to act as a method of immobilization. Casts can be made for the entire body, as for spinal injuries, for any portion of the body (spica cast), or for just the extremities.

Materials

There are many materials currently used in the manufacture of casts, but plaster of paris is still the most common in orthopaedics. In addition to being the most widely used, it is the cheapest material available. It has the advantage of being easily handled, with the ability to conform completely too any surface. Its strength capabilities are more than adequate for small animal application. Other types of casting material are thermal plastics, fiberglass, and polyurethane-impregnated cotton polyester. All of these splinting materials have special advantages along with certain disadvantages.

Plaster of Paris application

1. The animal is sedated and restrained in lateral recumbency with the affected limb uppermost.
2. The affected limb including foot is cleaned and dried.
3. Any wound, if present, should be cleaned, debried, covered with antiseptic dressing and bandage.
4. After reduction of the fracture boric acid powder liberally applied to the limb.
5. The coronary band, dew claws, and other bony prominence should be adequately padded with cotton.
6. Apply bandage to cover the layer of cotton.
7. POP deep in luck warm water (Temp. 30-35 °C recommended) for moistening the plaster roll. If the water is too hot, the cast will set too rapidly and will not allow time to construct a good cast in one solid unit. Too cold water causes delay in the setting time thus prolonging the period of restraint of the animal.

8. Plaster rolls should be submerged completely in water using both hands till air bubbles stop emerging.

9. The rolls should be gently squeezed to remove excess water.

10. When the cast is being applied, it is important not to create wrinkles or creases in the initial layers to avoid pressure sores.

11. The plaster bandage should be applied spirally over the limb, running either from top to bottom or bottom to top, so that one roll of the material forms a thin layer at entire cast site, rather than being wrapped at one place.

12. Each turn of the plaster bandage should overlap previous turn by half width and may be folded on itself to change the direction.

13. The cast is contoured to the limb by folding, twisting or tucking as the POP bandages are unrolled.

Bandage care

Keep bandage/splint clean and dry.

Observe digits for coolness/swelling.

Observe for evidence of self mutilation/foul odour (If problems noted, remove and reassess).

Observe for evidence of pressure sores.

Keep bandage/splint intact for 3-4 weeks.

Chapter 47

Thomas Splint and Robert Jones Bandage

Thomas Splint

The Schroeder-Thomas splint is a traction device that has proved useful in the treatment of fractures in small animals.

Indications

- To immobilize any fracture distal to the mid femur or mid humerus.
- To immobilization of joints distal to the knee and the elbow.

Preparation

The Schroeder-Thomas splint is custom made to each animal, and its shape changes in relation to the extremity injured and the purpose for which the splint is designed. In the hind leg the Schroeder-Thomas splint can be useful in immobilizing distal femoral or tibial fractures. Because most femoral fractures are usually stabilized by other means, the construction of the Schroeder-Thomas splint will be described for use in tibial fractures.

To make a Schroeder-Thomas splint it is necessary to have adequate supplies of materials like aluminium road, cotton bandage, splint mold, adhesive tape etc. The frame of the splint is made of aluminum rods. The external frame should be sufficiently stiff that it will not bend and deform when used by the animal in an appropriate manner. The first important component to manufacture for the splint is the upper ring, which encompasses the thigh. The diameter of this ring can be determined by measuring the distance between the tip of the wing of the ilium and the point of the ischium. The ring should be constructed in a round fashion, which can usually be done by fashioning the rod around an appropriate mold. These molds are available commercially or can be made in a large variety of sizes by using round wooden circles of 3/4 in diameter wood bolted together in sequence. Once the ring has been fashioned, the splint should be fitted to the animal. By lifting the leg it can be seen that the round splint will not conform to the medial side in the groin area. It is important, therefore, to bend the ring in an approximately 45 angle and flatten the ring so that it will conform to the dog's body. For this, the lower portion of the ring is placed in a vice, and the bend is made approximately half way up the cranial border of the ring and approximately 1/3 of the way up the caudal border of the ring. This portion of the ring is then flattened and padded. Very little padding is needed. Tape is usually applied to the ring so that the sticky side is facing outward and a thin strip of cotton padding is wrapped around the tape. The tape is then reversed and the cotton is covered to protect it from becoming soiled and moist. The length of the Schroeder-Thomas splint is determined by placing the dog's leg in a normal standing position; a right-angle bend is made at the distal end of the splint approximately 1 inch longer than the length of the dog's leg. It is important not to hyperextend the dog's leg when making this measurement; it should be in a normal position so that the splint will not be too long for the dog when walking. Since the Schroeder-Thomas splint is a traction device, it is important that its width be sufficient to allow traction of the leg so that they will not contact the device itself. Bending of the bar in the cranial surface of the Schroeder-Thomas splint would be at the level of the knee and again at the level of the hock. It is important that this to be done in a way that allows the padding to be appropriately placed.

Following construction of the splint, the outside of the aluminum frame is covered with adhesive tape to prevent slippage of the traction slings before they are applied.

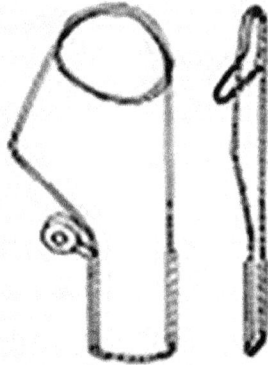

Figure 47.1: A pelvic limb Schroeder-Thomas splint.

When applying the Schroeder-Thomas splint to the hind leg, it is important to know for what purpose it is being applied. The shape of the splint is basically the same for any area, but traction should always be applied to the bone that is fractured or requires immobilization. Following the application of the splint to the dog's foot by the cranial and caudal strips of tape, the hock joint is stabilized with the first band of combine roll, which is approximately the length of this splint. The combine roll is looped over the posterior aspect of the bar underneath or medial to the tarsus and the entire roll is brought around laterally so that the hock is pulled back into position. The hock is brought back so it touches the metal bar. The combine roll is continued around through the splint to provide medial support and is then pulled to tension and secured with tape. At this point reduction of the fracture is accomplished and a second piece of combine roll, which is approximately 1.5 to 2 times the length of the splint, is used to secure the femur in a cranial position in relation to the splint. In this case the procedure followed at the distal hock is repeated in reverse so that the femur is pulled forward to the bar, but after the combine roll has passed through the splint it then provides medial support to the tibial area by constant figure-of-eight motions within the splint. Following tightening of the combine roll and taping it in place, the fracture is checked for stability. It is important that the ring of the Schroeder- Thomas splint be in contact with the groin area and not allows motion at the fracture site. Depending on the swelling adjust the splint the following day and every three or four days thereafter.

The traction itself will not displace the fracture but will provide adequate tension on the already contracted musculature, thereby providing stability at the fracture site. When applying a Schroeder-Thomas splint for fracture of the tibia, the bands should go around the hock joint first and then above the femur area to provide traction of the tibia. If, in fact, the fracture is of the femur, the bands should go around the hock joint and then around the proximal tibia or distal femur to provide stability and traction in the femur. The traction exerted in the femur is provided between the bar under the groin and the uppermost traction band.

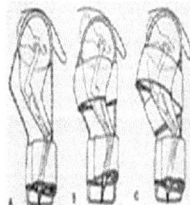

Figure 47.2: Application of a Schroeder-Thomas splint. (A) The bottom sling is placed first, as shown. Following completion, the combine roll material is taped in place. (B) The process is reversed to apply the top combine roll to pull the femur forward, thereby applying traction to the tibia. (c) Medial support is applied to the tibia by continuation of the bandage medial to the tibia.

This Schroeder-Thomas splint applied on the front leg looks considerably different than on the back leg. The use of the Schroeder-Thomas on the front leg for distal humeral fractures, elbow fractures, or radial and ulnar fractures may allow for considerable change in the form that the splint takes. For mid shaft humeral fractures, which are about the upper limit for use of this device, the splint will be relatively straight. As the fracture becomes more distal, the positional shape of the splint will become more and more that of a right angle as the result of the relationship of the fractured fragments to the pull of the muscles that surround them. For midshaft fractures, direct traction on the leg will help reduce and immobilize the fracture fragments. When fractures occur at the distal end of the humerus, the extensors of the carpus and forepaw will rotate the distal fragment cranially. In this instance traction on the leg will produce a misalignment of the fractured humerus. The Schroeder-Thomas splint is made at a 90° angle, thereby allowing the fracture ends to be united in a more normal fashion. To make a Schroeder-Thomas splint for the front leg, the size of the ring is usually determined by the length of the scapular spine. The ring is flattened considerably into a large oval, and the distal aspect of the ring is bent medially to a 30 to 45 angle with the oval. The splint is padded, as it is in the back leg, and then bent according to the shape of the fracture. When bending the splint to the required shape it is important to seat the splint closely under the axilla while putting the elbow distally. The caudal bar of the splint should be bent at the elbow approximately 1 to 2 inches beyond the distal aspect of the elbow, and the cranial bar bent proximally 1 to 2 inches proximal to the elbow joint. This can be either a gentle bend, as in a midshaft fracture or a right-angle bend, as in a distal humeral fracture. The length of the splint is determined by extending the leg in a relaxed manner so that the end of the splint will coincide with the end of the toe when extended to the splint. The foot is attached to the splint in the same manner as described for the hind foot, using tape on the cranial and caudal aspect of the paw. In the front leg, the wraps (combine roll) are applied first at the level of the elbow, pulling the humerus backward and second at the level of the carpus, pulling it forward. This allows for a leverage effect that can increase the tension in the radius, ulna, or humerus when the second wrap is applied. Following the wraps the Schroeder-Thomas splint can be covered again with a stockinette. Adjustments are provided on the same time schedule as with the hind-leg Schroeder-Thomas splint.

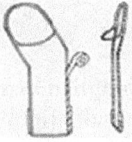

Figure 47.3: The front-leg Schroeder-Thomas splint would assume this shape for a midhumeral fracture

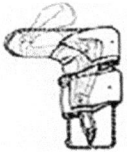

Figure 47.4: A right-angled Schroeder-Thomas splint. The first combine roll traction bandage is applied to the elbow region. The second traction bandage uses the first as a fulcrum and applies additional gentle traction to the humerus.

Robert Jones Bandage

This bulky bandage for immobilization of an extremity, first used by Sir Robert Jones, was popularized in veterinary medicine by R.B. Hohn. The principle involved in the fixation is that of a large bulky dressing wrapped very tightly to the extremity, providing supreme comfort and relative immobility of the injured site.

Indications

- Temporary dressing for immobilization of fractures and is especially useful for traumatized extremities with a great deal of swelling or edema.

- To partially immobilizing joints following reconstructive surgery of the knee, such as cruciate or patella surgery.

Application

The Robert Jones dressing is applied using absorbent cotton roll. Following application of a stirrup on the dorsal and ventral surfaces of the foot, one-pound rolls of cotton are wrapped firmly around the extremity such that approximately two rolls would be used in an average 40 to 50   pound dog. This bulky bandage is then wrapped with elastic gauze so that it is firmly adherent to the leg. Further compression of the bandage is accomplished with the use of elastic tape. The dressing should be applied quite firmly so that the finished configuration sounds like a ripe watermelon when tapped with a finger. The bandage can be left on for 10 days, at which time it should be changed if it is still needed. Loosening of the bandage occurs over this 10-day period, and to a great extent immobility is lost. This dressing is sometimes used following cast or splint removal, especially in tendon surgery, to allow gradual partial return to weight bearing. As the splint loosens over the 10-day period, weight bearing is increased slowly.

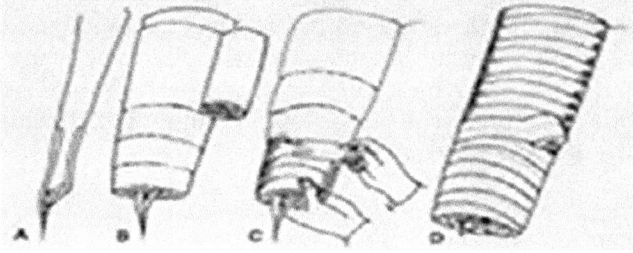

Figure 47.5: Application of a Robert Jones Bandage. (A) The tape stirrup is applied to the foot before the bandage is started. (B) Cotton roll is wrapped around a forelimb after the application of tape stirrup. (C) Elastic gauze is then applied to firmly bind the cotton to the leg. (D) Elastic tape is then used to complete the dressing.

Chapter 48

Intramedullary Pinning in Dogs

Intramedullary pinning is indicated for diaphyseal fracture of long bones, irregular transverse and short oblique fracture, spiral and comminuted fracture with ancillary fixation. It is simple, inexpensive technique. The disadvantage of the technique is there is no rotational stability of the fracture fragments.

Surgical techniques

A. Retrograde technique for femur fracture

The surgical site was shaved and scrubbed with povidone iodine scrub solution. In the operating room, the dog was positioned in lateral recumbency with the affected limb above and a sterile surgical scrub was carried out. The operating site was covered by draped to prevent surface contamination. The fracture site was approached by making a craniolateral incision. A linear skin incision was made along a line extending from the trochanter major to the lateral surface of the patella. The subcutaneous tissues were divided bluntly and tensor fascia lata was exposed. The attachments of the cranial border of the biceps femoris muscle with tensor fascia lata were severed to expose the vastus lateralis muscle cranially and biceps femoris muscle caudally. The belly of the biceps femoris muscle was reflected caudally and vastus lateralis and fascia lata were reflected cranially. The intermuscular septum between the two muscles was divided to expose the fractured.

Using retractors, the fractured fragments were exposed. Minimal separation of attached soft tissues was done. The ends of the fragments were debrided using a bone cutter and cleaned with a periosteal elevator. Bone fragments with no soft tissue attachments were removed. Soft callus at the fracture site was left undisturbed. Fracture reduction was carried out by using pointed reduction forceps.

Steinmann pin is inserted from the fracture site into the medullary canal of the proximal fragment with a steady pressure and back and forth quarter turns of the pin chuck. The pin is advanced up the medullary cavity till it comes out of the trochanteric fossa and out of skin. The pin chuck is disengaged and applied to the pin protruding from the skin. The pin is withdrawn slowly, again by making $1/4^{th}$ turn of the wrist, till its end is level with the distal end (Fracture end) of the proximal segment. Fracture is reduced aligned and held in the normal position. Pin chuck is advanced so as to send the pin down the medullary cavity of the distal segment, where it is seated in the metaphysis area. The pin setting is evaluated by radiography. The excess pin, protruding from the skin at trochanteric fossa is cut with pin cutter as close as possible and pushed under the skin. Extreme caution is taken to avoid penetration of distal/adjacent joint surface. The surgical wound is closed by routine manner.

B. Normograde technique

The pin was driven through the trochanteric fossa of the femur bone passing from the proximal to the distal fragment transversing the fracture line and impacting in the metaphysis of the opposing fragment. While inserting the pin, the distal fragment was angled slightly caudally to allow the deeper pin insertion in the cancellous bone of distal metaphysis to achieve proper point fixations. The pin was cut leaving 5-10 mm protruding to allow for removal after complete healing of the fracture.

Chapter 49

Neurological Examination, Diagnostic Nerve Block and Neurectomy

A neurological examination is the assessment of sensory neuron and motor responses, especially reflexes, to determine whether the nervous system is impaired.

A neurologic examination evaluates

1) The cranial nerves,

2) The gait, or walk,

3) The neck and front legs, and

4) The torso, hind legs, anus, and tail

The objective of a neurological exam is three fold

1. To identify an abnormality in the nervous system.

2. To differentiated peripheral from central nervous system lesions.

3. To establish internal consistency.

Instrumentation

The equipments are eye penlight, a percussion hammer and a pair of hemostatic forceps.

Physical examination

A. Visual system

Eye - Vision and pupil reflex

Cojuctivitis - Distemper, rabies

Corneal edema - Adenovirus infection

Corneal ulcers - Leads to tear production and inability to close of eyelid due to facial nerve disease

Chorioretinitis - In fungal, distemper, toxoplasmosis

Anterior uveitis – feline infectious peritonitis, toxoplasmosis, lymphosarcoma-in cat

B. Respiratory System

Nasal discharge

Nasal tumor

Larynx and pharynx

Pulmonary disease

C. Cardiovascular System

Heart failure

Cyanosis

D. Gastrointestinal system

Vomiting, diarrhea and weight loss.

Liver disorder - hepatic encephalopathy.

Pancreatic beta - cell neoplasia, hypoglycemia-seizures.

Diabetes mellitus.

E. Hemolymphatic system

Anemic condition

Enlarge lymph node

Petechiae and ecchymoses on skin and mucous membrane –bleeding disorder

F. Urinary system

Palpation and clinicopathological test

G. Reproductive system

Mammary adenocarcinoma, prostatic adenocarcinoma, pyometra

H. Skeletal system

Cranium and vertebrae examination for fracture, mass develop, other malformation

Neurological examination

A. Evaluation of the head

- History of seizures? Yes or No.
- Endocrinopathies - Polyuria, polydipsia, polyphagia.
- Head posture.
- Head coordination.
- Cranial nerves examination.

B. Evaluation of gait and strength

Evaluation of the gait by observing walks, runs, turns steps to the side and backs up. Signs of dysfunction include circling, weakness or complete paralysis of any limbs, falling, stumbling, rolling or loss of co-ordination.

C. Evaluation of forelimbs and neck

- Wheelbarrow
- Hopping
- Placing
- Proprioception
- Extensor strength
- Biceps reflex
- Triceps reflex
- Extensor carpi radialis

- Flexor reflex
- Crossed extension
- Deep pain
- Babinski sign
- Superficial sensation
- Neck pain
- Muscle atrophy

D. Evaluation of rear limbs, tail and anus

- Wheelbarrow.
- Placing.
- Proprioception.
- Extensor strength.
- Patellar reflex.
- Cranial tibial reflex.
- Gastrocnemius reflex.
- Flexor reflex.
- Crossed extension

- Hopping
- Deep pain.
- Babinski sign.
- Anal reflex.
- Tail response.
- Panniculus.
- Sensory level.
- Muscle atrophy.

Wheelbarrow– The hind limb lifted and supported, forcing to walk forward entirely on its front limbs.

Hopping– Both hind limbs and one forelimb are lifted and supported, so animal is relying on one forelimb.

Placing– Animal lifted and supported under thorax and abdomen and advanced toward table.

Proprioception– Standing the forelimb knuckled over at paw and observing ability of the animal to correct this abnormal position.

Babinski sign– Medial to lateral upward stroking of the metacarpal bone by percussion hammer.

Ancillary tests

The most common ancillary tests includes

1. X-rays of the cervical spine.
2. Myelogram.
3. Cerebrospinal fluid analysis.

X-Rays

The portions of the horse's body that are easily accessible to X-rays include the skull and the cervical spine. Other areas are too thick for even the most penetrating X-ray beam or require general anaesthesia to obtain the correct exposure.

Myelogram

The myelogram must be done under general anaesthesia. In this procedure, X-rays of the horse's spine are taken while a contrast agent is placed in the space surrounding the spinal cord. This does involve some risk to the horse, as the contrast agent must be placed into the atlanto-occipital space - a little bit behind the level of the horse's ears. There is a portion of the brain at this area, so the veterinarian must be very careful not to hit the brain with the needle that is used to place the contrast agent into the space. After the contrast agent is placed, X-rays are taken while the neck is manipulated in order to see if the spinal cord becomes pinched during these maneuvers - thus confirming a diagnosis of Wobbler's Syndrome.

Cerebrospinal fluid analysis

In this procedure, a small amount of fluid is removed from the area surrounding the spinal cord. This can be done in the standing, sedated horse, from the lumbosacral space (roughly at the level of the highest point of the croup) or in the anaesthetized horse from the atlanto-occipital space. It is less risky to the horse to retrieve the fluid from the lumbosacral space, but more risky to the person performing the maneuver. The fluid can be analyzed for protein, cells, or evidence of diseases such as equine protozoal myeloencephalopathy (EPM).

Other, less common ancillary tests include the EEG, which measures the electrical activity of the brain or brain waves, the electromyelogram, which tells us about the electrical activity of muscle cells and the nerves that control those cells. Nerve conduction tests, which tell us about the way that signals, are going through peripheral nerves. Computed tomography (CT scan), which can give us a more detailed picture of the brain, skull, vertebrae and spinal cord than an X-ray can.

Diagnostic Nerve Block in Equine

Regional nerve block or more commonly nerve block is a general term used to refer to the injection of local anaesthetic onto or near nerves for temporary control of pain. It can also be used as a diagnostic tool to identify specific nerves as pain generators. Permanent nerve block can be produced by destruction of nerve tissue.

Methods

Temporary nerve blocks are achieved by combining a local anaesthetic with epinephrine, a steroid, and/or opioids. Epinephrine produces constriction of the blood vessels which delays the diffusion of the anaesthetic. Steroids can help to reduce inflammation. Opioids are painkillers. Injection nerve blocks can be either single treatments, multiple injections over a period of time or continuous infusions. A continuous peripheral nerve block can be introduced into a limb undergoing surgery.

Permanent nerve block can be effected using other drugs or methods including alcohol or phenol to selectively destroy nerve tissue, cryoanalgesia to freeze nerves and radiofrequency ablation to destroy nerve tissue using heat.

Nerve blocks are sterile procedures that are usually performed in an out patient facility or hospital. The procedure can be performed with the help of ultrasound or fluoroscopy. Use of any one of these imaging modalities enables the physician to view the placement of the needle. A probe positioning system can be used to hold the ultrasound transducer steady.

Types

Certain nerve blocks are commonly used in horse. Each block involves the palmar nerve or its branches which are located in the forelimb.

Palmar digital nerve block - The palmar digital nerves (formerly known as the posterior digital nerves) run down the back of the pastern, one on each side of the deep flexor tendon. These nerves provide feeling to the back third of the horse's foot including:

- Sensitive tissues of the hoof wall, sole and frog.
- Coronet and heel bulbs.
- Lower half of the pastern (back part only).

Deeper structures of the foot (digital cushion, back third of the coffin bone, lateral cartilages, navicular bone and bursa, deep flexor tendon and its sheath).

This block is one of the technique used to diagnose navicular disease because the navicular bone and associated structures are typically desensitized by the block may be contributing to the lameness.

Low palmar nerve block - The low palmar (also known as the abaxial sesamoidian) block to desensitizes the palmar nerves. Blocking both the medial and lateral palmar nerves near the base of the sesamoid bones desensitizes the entire foot and at least half of the pastern. Blocking above the sesamoid bones may desensitize part of the fetlock and sesamoid bones with variable success.

4-point nerve block - The 4-point nerve block involves the two palmar nerves and the palmar metacarpal nerves. Blocking these four nerves desensitizes the foot, pastern, and entire fetlock joint, including the sesamoid bones.

Neurectomy

Neurectomy is employed mostly in horses as a palliative last resource to prolong the utility of working horses in certain incurable limb affections.

A. Median Neurectomy

Anaesthesia and Control

Median nerve block after deep sedation. In lateral recumbency with the affected limb below.

Site

The most superficial point immediately below the medial radial tuberosity, in the groove between the posterior border of radius and the flexor carpi radialis muscle.

Surgical technique

A 2" incision is made at the site along the posterior border of the radius. The tough fascia is cut and the groove, as mentioned above, is exposed. The median nerve lies superficially over artery and vein. The nerve is raised above the incision with the help of a tenaculum. The nerve is held with an artery forceps at the proximal end. A " to ½" piece of the nerve is removed below the artery forceps. Crushing of the cut end of the nerve is essential to avoid neuroma formation. The skin wound is approximated with interrupted sutures using cotton thread.

Post-operative care: The sutures are removed on 7th or 8th post-operative day.

B. Ulnar Neurectomy

Anaesthesia and Control

Ulnar nerve block after deep sedation. Lateral recumbency with the affected limb above.

Site

About 4" above the upper border of accessory carpal bone along a line joining the point of elbow.

Surgical technique

A2" long incision is made at the site. The aponeurosis of flexor muscles is cut. The nerve is quite superficial and is revealed as a thin, wavy, whitish cord-like structure. A piece of nerve is cut as described in the procedure of median neurectomy. The skin edges approximated with interrupted sutures using cotton thread.

Post-operative care: The sutures are removed on 7th or 8th post-operative day.

C. Anterior Tibial Neurectomy

Anaesthesia and Control

Local infiltration at the site after deep sedation. Lateral recumbency with the affected limb upwards.

Site

A 2" below and behind the lateral tuberosity of tibia or on the lateral aspect of the leg about 6" above the hock, in the groove between long and lateral digital extensor muscles.

Surgical technique

A 2" incision is made through skin and subcutaneous tissue at the site. The aponeurotic sheath is cut-open and the nerve is visible as a distinct white cord in the groove formed between the long and lateral digital extensor muscles. The nerve is divided on the, lines as described in median neurectomy. The skin is approximated by interrupted sutures.

Post-operative care: The sutures are removed on 7th or 8th post-operative day.

D. Posterior Tibial Neurectomy

Anaesthesia and Control

Local infiltration at the site after deep sedation. Lateral recumbency with the affected limb below.

Site

On the medial aspect of the leg, about a hand breadth above the point of hock and ½" in front of tendoachilles.

Surgical technique

A 1-1½" skin incision is made along the course of the nerve. The aponeurosis covering the nerve is cut to expose it. Apiece of nerve is removed as described for median neurectomy.

Post-operative care: The sutures are removed on 7th or 8th post-operative day.

Chapter 50

Claw Trimming

A cow with sore feet may realize losses in milk production, diminished breeding efficiency and decreased salvage value in the case of severe lameness. A 45° angle of the hoof is required for the greatest amount of shock absorption. Toes on each hoof should be about equal length, with all four feet approximately the same shape. The hind feet are likely to get longer on the toes than the front feet, and may need trimming more often. Trim the feet of cows that show excessive hoof growth or lameness. Use a couple of hoof knives, a rasp and hoof nippers, when the cow is restrained properly, begin with the hoof knife. It should remove very little tissue from the heels, but may take more as required to pull towards the toes.

The goal is to get the length in proper proportion to the foot shape desired. Cutting should be started from the underside of the hoof. Again, take small bites at a time to prevent injure of the foot. The finished hoof should be slightly concave so most of the weight is supported by the outer horny wall. The hoof should set flat when placed on the ground. A common mistake is to trim too much from the toe, leaving a rounded bottom to the hoof. Finish the hoof by rasping or sanding the rough areas.

Post operative care

Keep cattle areas dry. Wet floors tend to keep the soles soft, so they are subject to more mechanical injuries and foot rot.

Use a copper sulfate foot bath to help control foot rot.

Allow the cow plenty of room to exercise so they wear feet down.

Don't turn freshly trimmed cows out on rough, frozen ground.

Use a well-balanced ration with an adequate amount of fiber.

Chapter 51

Tenetomy and Tenecotomy

Plantar Tenotomy

Indications

Contracted tendon/knuckling.

Anaesthesia and Control

Local infiltration at the site or retrograde intravenous analgesia. Animal should be restraint in lateral recumbency.

Site

Fore limb: Middle of the metacarpal on the medial aspect.

Hind limb: Middle of the metatarsal on the lateral aspect.

Surgical technique

A 2" incision is taken along the anterior border of the flexor tendons. The skin is undermined. The subcutaneous fascia is cut to expose the flexor tendons. With the help of a tenaculum the flexor tendons are raised to the incision. The blood vessels lying along the anterior border of the deep digital flexor tendons should be avoided. Depending upon the severity of contraction of the tendons either only the superficial flexor tendon or both the superficial and deep digital flexor tendons are divided. Extension of the fetlock facilitates the division of the tendons. An antibiotic powder is sprinkled in the wound and the skin edges are approximated by interrupted sutures using cotton thread. After sealing of the wound the area is bandaged. The limb is immobilized by plaster of paris bandage from knee/hock downwards.

Post-operative care: After 15 days the plaster cast is removed. Massage of the limb and exercise is advised.

Gastrocnemius Tenectomy in Bullock

Indication

To relieve spastic paresis.

Surgical Anatomy

Achilles tendon is formed by twisting of three tendons and two calcaneal tendinous insertions *viz.*, superficial and deep tendons of gastrocnemius, superficial digital flexor tendon as well as calcaneal tendons of semitendinosus (covering latero-posteriorly) and biceps femoris (covering antero-medially).

Anaesthesia and Control

Sedation is achieved by injecting xylazine and local infiltration at the site of skin incision and deeply in and around the Achilles tendon. Animal is restrained in lateral recumbency keeping the affected limb above.

Site

Antero-lateral border of the Achilles tendon above the calcaneus (point of hock).

Surgical technique

A linear 8 cm long skin incision is made through the skin and subcutaneous tissues over antero-lateral border of the Achilles tendon, starting 3 cm above the point of hock. The calcaneal tendinous covering is incised parallel to the oblique depression present between the tendons of superficial digital flexor and medial head of gastrocnemius muscle. Through this incision superficial tendon of the gastrocnemius muscle along with the outer calcaneal covering elevated by a long curved artery forceps and transacted at two points about 4 cm apart. The deep tendon of gastrocnemius muscle placed cranio-medially is identified and its covering is incised longitudinally. Deep tendon of gastrocnemius is then exteriorised from its fibrous calcaneal sheath, transected at two points and a 3 cm piece is removed. The superficial digital flexor tendon and deep tendinous calcaneal covering is kept intact. Bleeding points are clamped and ligated. The subcutaneous tissues are sutured with placing a simple continuous layer of chromic catgut No.1 and skin edges with simple interrupted sutures using nylon filaments.

Allow the animal to move around loosely during post-operative period and start light work only after one month. In bilateral cases, second operation may be advised after complete recovery.

The traditional method of gastrocnemius tenotomy (Gotzes technique) consisting of resecting superficial gastrocnemius tendon completely and superficial digital flexor tendon partially, has well known post-operative complications like dropped hock, recurrence and sometimes no improvement in the condition whereas with the modified technique these complications are usually not encountered.

Lateral Digital Extensor Tenoctomy in Equine

Indication

To correct stringhalt.

Surgical Anatomy

Resection of the tendon and muscle belly leads to partial or even complete relief of the condition. The lateral digital extensor muscle originates at the collateral ligament of the stifle, fibula and lateral fibula; it proceeds distal, lateral to the tibia and enters to the tendon sheath just caudal to the lateral malleolus of the tibia.

Anaesthesia

General anaesthesia if large belly is to be removed, local anaesthesia is enough it is small muscle is to be involved. Local anaesthesia to be injected 2 cm above the lateral malleolus of the tibia directly into the muscle belly of the lateral digital extensor. The second injection of local anaesthetic solutions should be injected in the area below the hock and above the lateral digital extensor tendon just before it joins the long digital extensor tendon.

Surgical technique

The distal incision is made over the lateral digital extensor tendon immediately proximal to its junction with the long digital extensor tendon. An incision is made directly over the tendon the tendon is exposed and isolated by dissecting bluntly beneath the tendon and elevating it using either curved Kelly forceps or Oschner forceps. Severing is done at the mid area. Subcutaneous tissue and skin is closed in the routine manner.

Bandaging and Post-operative care should be done for 2-3 weeks or until completely heals.

Chapter 52

Dew Claw Removal and Amputation of Digit

Dew claw removal

Routinely medial hind claw is removed in cattle.

Indication

Prevention of self induced teat injuries.

Anaesthesia and Control

Anaesthesia is achieved by local infiltration or ring block or dorsal metatarsal vein injection following tourniquet application. Sedation with xylazine may be useful. Animal should be restraint in lateral recumbency.

Procedure

It is usually performed bi-laterally in calves but it can be unilateral or bilateral in adults. In calves heavy serrated scissors may be sufficient to remove the claw, where as sterile barnes or gouge –type dehorner works very well in adult cattle. Skin around the medial dew claw is clipped and surgically prepared. The animal should be restrained and the limb to operate should be raised. Following removal antiseptic dressing and bandage is applied and removed after 1 week.

Amputation of Digit

Indications

1. Crush wound the digit.
2. Foul-in-foot (foot rot).
3. Severe dermatitis (gangrenous dermatitis).

Anaesthesia and Control

Anaesthesia can be achieved by digital nerve block under tranquillization or retrograde intravenous anaesthesia or general anaesthesia. Animal should be restraint in lateral recumbency.

Site

An inverted 'T' shaped incision between the fetlock and coronet keeping the coronary band intact.

Surgical technique

A vertical incision is made on the lateral or medial face (depending on the digit to be amputated) of the fetlock to the coronet. Another incision is made around the coronet slightly above the coronary band. This result into an inverted 'T' shaped incision. The skin is flapped so as to expose the pastern joint. The digital vessels are ligated as high above as possible. The pastern joint is disarticulated, the tendons and ligaments are cut and the digit is removed. The exposed articular cartilage is rasped. The skin flaps are approximated with interrupted sutures leaving a slight space lower down for drainage. To control bleeding preferably the pouch is packed with sterile gauze. The limb is bandaged inclusive of the fetlock.

Post-operative care- On the next day of operation the sterile gauze is removed. The clots and dead tissues are removed. Some antiseptic ointment or antibiotic ointment is smeared in the pouch and the limb is bandaged. Further, the wound is daily dressed. The sutures are removed on 8th or 10th postoperative day.

Chapter 53

Patellar Luxation in Canine

Medial Patellar Luxation

A luxation of the patella is a common occurrence in small and toy breed dogs. Mild patella luxation may be managed conservatively, but more severe patella luxation should be treated surgically.

The techniques to correct the luxations may be divided in three groups: deepening of the trochlea, realignment of the quadriceps muscles over the trochlea and soft tissue techniques to reestablish appropriate soft tissue tension around the joint.

Anaesthesia and Control

General anaesthesia and lateral recumbency with affected limb below or dorsal recumbancy.

Preparation

The affected pelvic limb is clipped from the dorsal and ventral midline to just distal to the hock joint. The cranial border of the clipped area is approximately 10-15 cm cranial to the greater trochanter and the caudal border about 2-3 cm medial to the ischiatic tuberosity. The dog is placed in dorsal recumbancy. The clipped area of the suspended, affected leg is further prepared for surgery.

Approach

➢ A medial skin incision, extending from just proximal and medial to the patella to the distal tibial tuberosity is made.

➢ A medial arthrotomy (Medial desmotomy).

Surgical correction patella luxation

First, the patella is medially luxated and a V-shaped recession sulcoplasty ("wedge") recession using an exacto saw blade and a sterile razor blade are made. In small dogs and cats, a one-sided razor blade works very well for this procedure.

In larger dogs an exacto saw may be used. After reduction of the patella, the quadriceps alignment and patellar stability are evaluated by rotating the stifle in medial and lateral direction ("wiggle test"). If the patella luxates, a tibial crest transposition should be performed by cutting the crest using an osteotome and mallet. Leave a periosteal attachment at the distal aspect of the tibial crest. Move the tibial crest to a prepared site on the lateral aspect of the tibia. Stabilize the crest temporarily with a bone reduction forceps. After reduction of the patella, the quadriceps alignment and patellar stability are evaluated by rotating the stifle in medial and lateral direction. If the patella still luxates, the tibial crest should be transposed in a more lateral position. If the patella is stable, stabilize the crest with 2 K-wires, going through the tibial crest towards the medial tibial plateau. Manually evaluate for penetration of the cortex by the pins and stop advancement immediately after palpation of the pins.

The unnecessary joint capsule on the lateral side of the patella is removed and closes the ensuing lateral parapatellar arthrotomy with a cruciate pattern. Now the medial parapatellar arthrotomy is addressed. Often closure of this atrhrotomy is not possible without putting undue tension on the patella. If this is the case, leave the joint capsule incision partly or completely open and cover the defect with either crural fascia or subcutaneous tissue.

The lateral and medial crural fascia is closed using a cruciate suture pattern. Subcutaneous and subcuticular layers are closed using a simple continuous suture pattern with buried knots. The skin is sutured using a cruciate pattern.

Post operative care

A modified Robert Jones bandage may be applied to prevent swelling. Restricted exercise for 6 weeks.

Extra-Capsular Repair of CCL Rupture

Introduction

A ruptured cranial cruciate ligament is one of the most commonly diagnosed orthopaedic conditions in dogs. The procedure consists of a surgical exploration of the joint and meniscectomy, and stifles stabilization. Much different stabilization is being used. The modified retinacular imbrication technique is routinely used to repair the CCL.

Preparation

The affected pelvic limb is clipped from the dorsal and ventral midline to just distal to the hock joint. The cranial border of the clipped area is approximately 15 cm cranial to the greater trochantor and the caudal border about 2-3 cm medial to the ischiatic tuberosity. The patient is positioned in dorsal recumbancy, and the surgical field is further prepared for surgery with the leg hanging.

Approach

> A medial skin incision is made from about 2-3 cm proximal and slightly medial to the patella, extending to the distal portion of the tibial tuberosity. Incise the subcutaneous until the crural fascia has been reached.

➢ Preparation for stabilization sutures

  ❖ Medial side

    An incision is made in the medial crural fascia just cranial to the caudal head of the Sartorius muscle, from the tibial plateau to just proximal to the medial fabella.

    The location of the fabella is confirmed by putting a hemostat under the fabella and then "wiggling" it.

    The muscles distal to the fabella are bluntly separated and an Army-Navy retractor is placed to create space for passing the suture.

  ❖ Lateral side

    An incision is made in the lateral crural fascia just cranial to the biceps femoris muscle, from the tibial plateau to just proximal to the lateral fabella.

    The location of the fabella is confirmed by putting a hemostat under the fabella and then "wiggling" it.

    The muscles distal to the fabella are bluntly separated and an Army-Navy retractor is placed to create space for passing the suture.

Then a medial parapatellar arthrotomy is performed.

➢ A 1 cm incision is made through the fibrous joint capsule at the level of the parapatellar fat pad, about 0.5-1 cm medial to the patellar tendon.

➢ While extending the stifle joint, one "leg" of blunt Mayo scissors are put in the parapatellar fat pad through the small incision, and pushed into the joint cavity in proximal direction.

➢ The patella is immediately luxated in lateral direction and hemorrhage from the joint capsule is controlled.

Joint exploratation

➢ The cranial and caudal cruciate ligaments are evaluated for pathology and if the cranial cruciate ligament is ruptured, it is debrided using a No. 15 blade.

➢ The joint is checked for drawer movement.

➢ The joint is further explored.

    Patella – check for cartilage erosions and osteophytes.

    Long digital extensor tendon – check for enthesopathy.

    Synovial membrane – evaluate for inflammation and take biopsy if indicated.

    Menisci

    • Medial meniscus most commonly affected because of its stable attachments.

- Hook hemostat behind tibial plateau and luxate the tibia forward and evaluate lateral and medial meniscus.
- A meniscus may be partially or completely removed, depending on the pathology.
- If a medial meniscectomy is performed, start by detaching the cranial pole of the meniscus from the parapatellar fat pad, following by transaction of the intermeniscal ligament.

The arthrotomy is closed using a cruciate pattern.

Stabilization of the joint

→ A hole is created in the proximal portion of the tibial tuberosity. First, the tibialis cranialis muscle in the area of the tibial tuberosity is elevated from the tibia (first incise, and then use periosteal elevator). Then a hole is created with a small Steinman pin. The more proximal and cranial the hole is, the better the suture plane direction will mimic the plane of the cranial cruciate ligament.

→ Then a suture is brought around the lateral fabella perpendicular to the long axis of the femur. In this way, the needle and suture go through the retinaculum between the fabella and the patella, and the origin of the gastrocnemius muscle, thus minimizing the chances that the suture slips "off" the fabella and becomes non-functional.

→ A suture is brought around the medial fabella perpendicular to the long axis of the femur. In this way, the needle and suture go through the retinaculum between the fabella and the patella, and the origin of the gastrocnemius muscle, thus minimizing the chances that the suture slips "off" the fabella and becomes non-functional.

→ Both sutures are passed through the hole in the proximal portion of the tibial tuberosity.

→ Tie sutures and put knots in the lateral and medial indentation adjacent to the patella.

Closure

→ The lateral and medial crural fascia is imbricated using a cruciate suture pattern. Make sure that the knots of the stabilization suture are covered well with soft tissue.

→ Subcutaneous and subcuticular layers are closed using a simple continuous suture pattern with buried knots.

→ The skin is sutured using a cruciate pattern.

Post operative care

- A modified Robert Jones bandage may be applied to prevent swelling.
- Confinement and restricted activity for 6 weeks.

Chapter 54

Upward Fixation of the Patella

Patellar fixation is one of the main functional disorders of the tibia-femoral-patellar articulation (knee joint) in cattle characterized by temporary or permanent dislocation of the patella from its normal position during locomotion. Such dislocation may be dorsal, lateral or medial, causing a dorsal, lateral or medial patellar fixation, respectively. The major potential factors for patellar fixation in cattle are nutrition deficiency, exploitation activity, breed and genetic tendency, external traumas, intense contraction of the crural triceps muscle and morphological changes of the trochlea and medial condyle of the femur.

Clinical sign

➢ Lameness after extended rest is the most typical sign.

➢ The fixation invokes slight extension of the limb, phalangeal flexion so that the animal drags the tip of the hoof.

➢ Leg "locks" in posterior phase of stride as the leg "unlocks" the limb is abducted as it advances to anterior portion of stride.

Medial Patellar Desmotomy

Indication

Chronic Subluxation of patella.

Anaesthesia and Control

Local infiltration at the site. Lateral recumbency with the affected limb below or in standing after animal secured in travis.

Site

The triangle formed by the anterior and medial tuberosity of tibia and patella itself. The skin incision is taken approximately over the anterior border of the medial straight ligament of the patella.

Surgical technique

There are two methods *viz.,* 1) Open and 2) Stab method.

Open Method: A 2" incision is taken along the anterior border of the medial straight ligament of the patella (there is a slight depression between the posterior border of the medial straight ligament and the medial border of the middle straight ligament of the patella). Alternately, the incision can be made along the posterior border of the medial straight ligament of patella. This can be achieved at a site 1/2" to 1" above and on a vertical plane with the anterior limit of the, condyle of the tibia. The skin is undermined and the medial straight ligament of patella is identified. A bistoury is held in a flat position and passed under the ligament. The sharp edge of the bistoury is turned towards the ligament and the ligament is severed with gentle sawing movement. A clear depression results on cutting the ligament. Some antibiotic powder is sprinkled in the depression and the skin is approximated with interrupted sutures using cotton thread.

Stab Method: In this method instead of taking a skin incision, the bistoury is introduced under ligament holding it in a flat position. The sharp edge is turned towards the ligament and severed. No suturing of the skin is necessary. Infusion of any antibiotic ointment into the wound through the small opening made by bistoury is beneficial.

Post-operative care: The wound is routinely dressed. The sutures are removed on 8th post operative day.

Chapter 55

Amputation of Limb

Indications

1. Irreparable injury.

2. Gangrene.

3. Malignant disease.

Anaesthesia and Control

Animal is controlled in lateral recumbency under general anaesthesia with the affected limb up.

Site

Fore limb- Lower third of the humerus limb.

Hind limb- Middle third of the femur above the stifle joint.

Surgical technique

A tourniquet is applied below the elbow or the stifle as the case may be. Elliptical skin incisions are made on the medial and lateral surface at the site chosen to obtain two flaps of skin, which will cover stump after amputation. The muscles are cut at the skin incision level. The bone is sawed off at the desired level. The tourniquet is loosened. The bleeding vessels are ligated and the nerves ends are crushed. The muscle flaps are sutured so as to cover the bony stump. The skin flaps are approximated by mattress sutures using cotton thread. The stump is bandaged after putting sufficient padding.

Post operative care

The wound is routinely dressed and bandaged. The sutures are removed on 10th post operative day.

Chapter 56

Physiotherapy

Physiotherapy deals with the treatment of diseases by physical methods. Rehabilitation means restoration of functional utility of affected parts. Physiotherapy accelerates tissue healing by encouraging normal physiological processes so that the function of affected part is restored faster. Physiotherapy helps to correct deformities, develops by paralysed muscles and makes joint movements more supple and prevent deforming tendencies.

Diathermy

Deep heat (Diathermy)

Tissue temperature can be increased to a depth of 3-5 cm or more without overheating subcutaneous tissue or skin. Produced by conversion of energy into heat, and may penetrate to deep structures such as ligaments, bones, muscles, and joint capsules. It includes ultrasound, shortwave diathermy and microwave diathermy.

Ultrasound (US)

Acoustic vibration with frequencies above the audible range (>20,000 Hz) can produce thermal (heating) and nonthermal (cavitation, acoustic streaming, and standing waves) effects.

Thermal effects

> Ultrasound interacts with skin, fat, and muscle during treatment. Heating occurs at all of these tissues as a result of beam attenuation and absorption. Its effect is more pronounced at tissue interfaces where sound transmission discontinuities occur.

> Ultrasound is absorbed and attenuated more in bone, followed by tendon, followed by skin, muscle, and fat.

> Absorption (heating) is greatest at the bone–muscle soft-tissue interface.

> Thermal effects include increased distensibility of collagen fibers.

Nonthermal effects

- ➤ Cavitation-produces gas bubbles in a sound field due to turbulence, which, by their forced oscillation and bursting, are capable of disrupting tissue.
- ➤ Acoustic streaming-unidirectional movement of compressible material or medium due to pressure asymmetries caused by US waves.
- ➤ Acoustic streaming and cavitation are associated with wound contraction and protein synthesis.

Ultrasound indications

- ➤ Bursitis.
- ➤ Tendinitis (calcific tendinitis).
- ➤ Musculoskeletal pain.
- ➤ Degenerative arthritis and contracture (adhesive capsulitis, shoulder periarthritis and hip contracture).
- ➤ Subacute trauma.

Contraindications

- ➤ Near brain, cervical ganglia, spine, laminectomy sites (can cause spinal-cord heating).
- ➤ Near heart, reproductive organs.
- ➤ Near pacemakers-may cause thermal or mechanical injury to the pacemaker.
- ➤ Near tumors.
- ➤ Gravid or menstruating uterus.
- ➤ At infection sites.
- ➤ Near to the eye.
- ➤ Skeletal immaturity-open epiphysis can be affected with decreased growth due to thermal injury.

Shortwave diathermy (SWD)

- ➤ Produces deep heating through the conversion of electromagnetic energy (radio waves) to thermal energy.
- ➤ The most commonly used frequency is 27.12 MHz.
- ➤ Provides deep heat to 4–5 cm depth, therefore is good for deep muscle.
- ➤ The heating pattern produced depends on the type of shortwave unit and water content and electrical properties of the tissue.

Microwave diathermy

- ➤ Conversion of electromagnetic energy (microwaves) to thermal energy.

> Microwaves do not penetrate tissues as deeply as US or SWD.

Indications

> Used to heat superficial muscles and joints, to speed the resolution of hematomas, and for local hyperthermia in cancer patients

> The lower frequency has a higher depth of penetration, and is better for muscle heating

Electrical Stimulation

Consists of transcutaneous electrical stimulation for muscles with or without intact pripheral nervous system, or central control.

When the electrical stimulation is used to provide functional use of paretic muscles, it is called FES (functional electrical stimulation) or FNS (functional neuromuscular stimulation). Multiple muscles can be activated in a coordinated fashion through the use of electrical stimulation to attain certain functional goals (ambulation, transfers).

Uses

> Maintains muscle mass after immobilization.

> FES prevents complications from immobility such as deep vein thrombosis, and osteoporosis.

> Strengthens muscles effects have been noted even without voluntary muscle action. Changes of type II muscle fibers into type I fibers are temporarily noted with the treatments.

> FES inhibits spasticity and muscle spasm.

> FES can be used for orthotic training and functional movement.

> Radiation

Infrared

Infrared penetrates 7 to 10 mm deep into the skin. Source of infrared must be kept 25 to 30 cms away from the part to be treated. Exposure of infrared light to the nacked eye directly must be avoided. Infrared light should be applied for short duration maximum up to 20 to 30 minutes. Careful observations are required to prevent burn injuries of the part being exposed.

Ultraviolet

It has wavelength of 2000–4000 A . Bactericidal wavelength is 2537 A . It can be produced by a small, hand held mercury or "cold quartz" lamp. It produces a non-thermal photochemical reaction with resultant alteration of DNA and cell proteins.

> Physiologic effects

> Bactericidal on motile bacteria.

> Increased vascularization of wound margins.

> Hyperplasia and exfoliation.

➢ Increased Vitamin D production.

➢ Excitation of calcium metabolism.

Indications

- For treatment of aseptic and septic wounds.

- Psoriasis treatment- utilizes Goeckerman's technique, where a coal-tar ointment is applied to the skin prior to UV treatment.

- Acne treatment.

- Treatment of folliculitis.

Massage

Pressure and stretching are provided in a rhythmic fashion to the soft tissues. Physiologic effects include: Reflexive, mechanical and psychological

Reflexive effects

- Reflex vasodilation with improvement in circulation.

- Decrease in pain by means of the gate control or release of endogenous opiates or – neurotransmitters.

- General relaxation.

- Increased perspiration.

Mechanical effects

- Assists in venous blood return from the periphery to the CNS.

- Increase lymphatic drainage.

- Decrease muscle tightness.

- Prevents or breaks adhesions in muscles, tendons and ligaments.

- Softens scars.

- Loosening of secretions.

Psychological effect

"Laying of hands" promotes a sense of general well-being.

There is no effect on the metabolism. Massage will not affect muscle strength, mass, or rate of atrophy of denervated muscle.

Common techniques of therapeutic massage

Classical massage

- Effleurage- Gliding movement of the skin without deep muscle movement; used for muscle relaxation.

- Petrissage- Kneading, to increase circulation and reduce edema.

- Tapotement- Percussion. Helps with desensitization, allows clearing of secretions, and improves circulation. Used for chest therapy in conjunction with postural drainage.

- Friction massage- Prevents adhesions in acute muscle injuries and breaks adhesions in subacute and chronic injuries. Also reduces local muscle spasm and decreases edema. It can be applied transverse or perpendicular to the muscle, tendon or ligament fibers.

- Soft tissue mobilization- Forceful massage of the fascia-muscle system. Massage is done with the fascia-muscle in a stretched position, rather than relaxed or shortened. Used for reduction of contractures.

- Myofascial release- Prolonged light pressure is applied in specific directions of the fascia system to stretch focal areas of muscle or fascial tightness.

- Accupressure- Finger pressure is applied over trigger points or acupuncture points to decrease pain.

Galvanic Current

Galvanic current electricity is employed for the diagnosis of certain nervous and muscular lesions (electrodiagnosis), and in the treatment of different affections (electrotherapy). For therapeutic purposes continuous current (galvanisation), induced currents (faradisation), and high-frequency current are employed. Galvanic current is preferred. The current should be feeble and should not cause pain. The electrodes may be placed so that the current travels the spinal cord longitudinally from the forehead or from the poll backwards towards the lumber region, or perpendicularly from the dorso lumber region towards the sternum or abdomen. Electricity does not have any curative effect on lesions but it simply counteracts certain especially muscular contractions and atrophy of the muscles. To act on the limbs one poll is applied on the spine at the level of cervical or lumbar region of the cord and other at the extremity of the limb. The current is applied for 5 to 6 minutes daily or at a longer interval.

Hydrotherapy

It is Useful in sub acute and chronic inflammation. It is used to hasten the suppurative process. It also has a vasodilatation effect and thus it increases phagocytosis. Heat or warm water fomentation must not be used in presence of infection as well as 24 to 48 hours after trauma.

Indications

Acute congestion, acute inflammation and lesions when there is no danger of death of tissues from diminished blood supply.

Effects and Methods

Normal temperature of skin is 68 °F to 86 °F and the temperature of cold water varies from 48 °F to 59 °F. Cold water when applied to part produces a stimulant and sedative effect. It causes vasoconstriction in the skin and subcutaneous tissue and slows down the process of nutrition. An anodyne effect is produced in painful inflammatory lesions as long as cold applications are continued. Hydrotherapy may be in the form of baths, lotions, compresses or continuous irrigation. The best results are obtained when water is at 59 °F.

Hot water application

Indications

Sub acute and chronic inflammation, septic inflammation in which vitality of tissues is lowered.

Effects

1. Hyperaemia: It causes increase in blood flow to the area where hot water is applied this causes increase in exudation and increase in phagocytosis.

2. Analgesia is produced through softening and relaxing the tissues.

Method of application

Bath and fomentations can be utilized for this purpose. The temperature of water may be gradually raised from 30 °F to 113 °F or even 122 °F without scalding. The hot water is an excellent method of treating inflammatory condition of the foot or lower part of the limb. When the lesion is septic, an antiseptic agent is added it. The bath is also very beneficial for inflammation affecting the hindquarters of the dog including the pelvis and abdominal organs. At a temperature 113 °F moist heat diminishes the resistance of tissues. To have best results hot applications must be frequently renewed, or the temperature of the water be maintained by adding occasionally more hot water. Cold and hot water applications may be used alternately with good results.

Cold therapy

Cold application is indicated for the treatment of acute and hyper acute inflammatory conditions. Pain, muscle spasm and tissues metabolism is generally reduced following cold applications. Cold application should be combined with compression and rest, for further limiting the swelling of the part. This treatment is used for 24 to 48 hours after trauma. Each application should last for 20 minutes, an average of one hour interval between two applications is normally recommended. Coldwater irrigation, ice application and cold pack applications are generally recommended for cold therapy.

Index